Stroke Book

STROKE BOOK

THE DIARY OF A BLINDSPOT

Jonathan Alexander

Fordham University Press

New York   2021

Fordham University Press has no responsibility for the persistence or accuracy of URLs for external or third-party Internet websites referred to in this publication and does not guarantee that any content on such websites is, or will remain, accurate or appropriate.

Fordham University Press also publishes its books in a variety of electronic formats. Some content that appears in print may not be available in electronic books.

Visit us online at www.fordhampress.com.

Library of Congress Cataloging-in-Publication Data

Names: Alexander, Jonathan, 1967– author.
Title: Stroke book : the diary of a blindspot / Jonathan Alexander.
Description: First edition. | New York : Fordham University Press, 2021. | Includes bibliographical references.
Identifiers: LCCN 2021027355 | ISBN 9780823297665 (hardback) | ISBN 9780823297689 (epub)
Subjects: LCSH: Alexander, Jonathan, 1967– –Health. | Cerebrovascular disease–Patients–Biography. | Retina–Blood-vessels–Diseases. | Blindness. | Homosexuality–Social aspects.
Classification: LCC RC388.5 .A435 2021 | DDC 616.8/10092 [B]–dc23
LC record available at https://lccn.loc.gov/2021027355

Printed in the United States of America
23 22 21   5 4 3 2 1
First edition

For Mack McCoy,
for the obvious reasons, and the less obvious too

Preface

This book emerged out of a health crisis in the summer of 2019, and a need to think and feel that crisis through my sexuality, my changing sense of dis/ability, and my experience of time. At a basic level, the book, initially drafted in the immediate aftermath of the crisis (a minor stroke), chronicles a very mortal encounter with time, with my recognition that we are never not beholden to time, even as we often refuse opportunities to confront the feelings and realities of our beholdenness. But it is also a recognition that *queer* time has its own rhythms, fluctuations, and perversities. I experienced–and continue to experience–my health crisis in very particular ways, ways that I cannot disentangle from my experiences in this culture as a queer person. This book is a refusal to engage in disentanglement.

Previous writers on illness and narrative have attempted to account for the various pressures when narrating health crises to collapse the specificity of the suffering individual into a generalized human condition. Arthur W. Frank, in *The Wounded Storyteller: Body, Illness, and Ethics,* writes that "the ill person who turns illness into story transforms fate into experience; the disease that sets the body apart from others becomes, in the story, the common bond of suffering that joins bodies in their shared vulnerability" (xix).[1] While we might have a "shared vulnerability" through our inevitable mortality, the distribution of vulnerabilities–such as those that lead to different temporal and spatial proximities to mortality–are not so evenly distributed. Different class, racial, and gendered subject positions are more or less proximate to illness and mortality, with, in this country for instance, the working class, the non-white, and women consistently more prone to certain kinds of diseases, as well as differential access to quality health care, than the economically secure, the white, and men. Queer people often experience psychic and somatic pressures that not only decrease their overall quality of life (whatever that obscure phrase might mean) but that can also lead to shorter life spans–and not just due to the ravages of HIV infection and suicide, though those have been two significant causes of death for many queer

---

1   Arthur W. Frank, *The Wounded Storyteller: Body, Illness, and Ethics* (1995; Chicago: University of Chicago Press, 2013).

people. As Andrew Durbin wrote in a review of the work of Hervé Guibert, who chronicled his death from AIDS in a series of powerful books, "Disease *is* conspiratorial, never egalitarian, always crawling along social fissures."

The problem for any writer is how to manifest such entanglements *formally*, in a form of writing that one has either to borrow or concoct, not only to document the experience one is having but, hopefully, to render it in such a way that a curious reader can catch a glimpse of both the experience of the writer and also the larger web of world that makes the particularity of a singular experience *more*–that is, a form that allows a reader to see how any singularity is always *multiple*, even if it doesn't seem to be so in the phenomenological experience of it.

At first, I will admit, the exigence of the *form* of this book began as an attempt to circumvent the narrative troping, the turning and twisting, that Susan Sontag famously identified as all but inevitable in the narration of illness. We are forever turning our lives into material for metaphor, for comparative assessment, for measuring ourselves against that which surrounds us, against that which also permeates us. In writing in the aftermath of my "incident," I wanted instead, for myself and then increasingly for others, a phenomenological account that

spoke to the *immediacy* of my experience. I wanted
to communicate the content of the experience
as experience. I wanted to try to set aside, as much
as I could, the voices in my head, the perverse
implantations, that were whispering, say, about
god's punishment, among many other things–
the voices that were trying to tell me I either
deserved what happened to me, or that it was
inevitable, or that it held the key to a larger set of
hidden meanings. I wanted at least to try.

I did not succeed, and what you hold in your
hands is the resulting failure. What I could not do
was suspend all of those voices. They *were*, after
all, a key part of the experience.

Another way to talk about the origin of *Stroke Book*
is to acknowledge that others have gone before
me, and no book is born out of nothingness.
Formally, this book began, not fully consciously
on my part, as a response to Sarah Manguso's
compelling and experimental memoir, *Ongoingness.*
Manguso's is a slim and powerful book that
tackles in its title and in its brief, aphoristic
narratives, most barely spanning a page, the
problem of phenomenological time under the
sign of illness–in her case, an obsessive anxiety
disorder. The author tells us how she poignantly
experienced her days as time slipping away from
her, so she kept a diary, obsessively filling it with

as much information as she could, in an attempt
to offer a proper and complete accounting of
her time. As Manguso worried neurotically over
what she was doing with her time and her life,
the diary, stretching to 800,000 words, didn't
lessen her anxiety; instead it started to exacerbate
it: "It led neither away from the previous day
nor toward the following day. It possessed no
form separate from the greater form, which
itself was almost formless–which itself was just
accumulation, just *day after day after day after day*"
(93).[2] Fortunately we don't have to wade through
those 800,000 words. The book *Ongoingness* isn't
the diary that she kept; it is rather, in the words
of the little book's subtitle, an accounting of *The
End of a Diary*.

Still, *Ongoingness* is a *kind* of diary, maybe a
meta–diary, a nearly chronological rendering of
the experience of writing an out–of–control diary.
Manguso recounts her struggle with anxiety,
with the anxiety of ongoingness and her need
to write through that anxiety–until she has a
baby. As she puts it, "Before the baby was born,
the diary allowed me to continue existing. It
literally constituted me. If I didn't write it, I wasn't
anything, but then the baby became a little boy

---

2   Sarah Manguso, *Ongoingness: The End of a Diary*
(Minneapolis: Graywolf Press, 2015).

who needed me more than I needed to write the
diary. He needed me more than I needed to write
about him" (84). Ultimately for Manguso the baby
does more than just break a neurotic fixation;
it obliterates time as a measure: "I used to exist
against the continuity of time. Then I became the
baby's continuity, a background of ongoing time
for him to live against" (53). Fearing she might be
misunderstood, Manguso explains further: "What
I'm saying is that I have become, in a way, inured
to the passage of time. I'm not really paying
attention to what's happening to me anymore–no
longer observing steadfastly the things that have
changed since yesterday" (69).

As an account of one mother's shifted
experience of time in relation to giving birth,
Ongoingness likely offers much that, in its
particulars of childbearing, is relatable to many
women. I am not a woman, so the experience is
not relatable to me, and I came, perhaps queerly,
to mistrust the narrative arc that bent, almost
inexorably, to fulfillment through reproduction,
to cure through the child. (I've likely read too
much Lee Edelman.) I kept asking myself after
having read the book, *what if one does not have a
child, or does not want a child? How does one understand
what to do with one's time when, all of a sudden, that
time seems potentially truncated, when one's mortality is*

made evident, and one does not have recourse to the child to sustain and extend oneself?

Thematically, Manguso couldn't help me. But *formally*, she did. As I began to write my text, my own obsessive diary, I approached my crisis much like Manguso did hers, most notably in my articulation of my experience, through short, diaristic bursts of text. Moreover, at a *material* level, Manguso's half pages, sometimes just a sentence, offered me a way to represent my damaged sight, the manifestation of my stroke. Through my right eye, my dominant eye, the one with which I read, I can now only see straight on, the lower left part of my vision grayed out, a blindspot. What once looked like a whole page of text now appears as partial, truncated. Manguso's partial pages presented me a possible model for visually depicting my new vision.

Even more, the bursts of text, some shorter, some longer, and their seemingly scattershot arrangement that nonetheless slowly builds toward an end, offered me a way to conceive of my diary as less a linear passage through time than a shifting, recursive, doubling back, reaching forward, and generally disturbed experience of time. If Manguso's formal approach helped her represent her anxious experience of the accumulation of time bending toward something generated (a child), I could potentially use a similar approach to capture my sense of fractured time, of time split open and made palpably finite while also bending back on itself, wondering what I have done to deserve this. What course, what path, what wrong turn on my temporal trajectory has led me to this moment, this bad stroke of luck?

But then, more positively, how might the half page help me see *differently* the days cut short, my sight *halved*—not just as a loss but as a *critical* gain, an *insight*? In the process of writing, I hoped to be able to show my now very *queered* sense of normative (both heteronormative and homonormative) time—a normative time that values a trajectory of bodily integrity and resistance to bodily disintegration, despite how inevitable such disintegration is. What writing through my health crisis offered me was an opportunity to begin to piece together scattered incidents, once seemingly remote occurrences, in an attempt to create a narrative of explanation, or meaningfulness, or even just survivability—but also of potential pleasure in the piecing together. In time, I came to feel how such piecing together of experience disrupts normative trajectories of health *and* also opens up possibilities for experiencing queer relations among the episodes of one's life.

I borrowed the idea of piecing, of stitching
together, from Maggie Nelson, who said that,
while writing *The Argonauts*, she would lay out her
various short passages (some narrative, others
more theoretical) on the floor, arranging and
rearranging them into a flow that made sense,
even if unexpectedly so. I found myself doing the
same, documenting in the form of the diary my
ongoing, unfolding experience in the aftermath
of the stroke, but then arranging and rearranging
bits and pieces to generate connections, some
even perverse and unexpected. As such, this
book is ultimately not a diary in any strict sense;
it is not even a chronological accounting. Yes, I
started *Stroke Book* in the immediate aftermath,
but I found myself dipping in and out of the
text, writing in linear time one day and then
circling back the next to fill in, augment,
contradict. As the text grew, further shifting and
rearranging seemed appropriate, and that process
itself became subject to its own backtrackings
and rearrangements of rearrangements. The
composing process became its own metaphor for
my experience of the crisis queerly–as a crisis that
was immediately experienced but also meditated
on and evocative of the past and memory and
also deranging of the past as well as my sense of
the present and its slippage into the future.

What kinds of connections does such a process
open up for a writer? Nelson is instructive here.
While *The Argonauts*, like Manguso's book, steadily
moves toward the arrival of her own child,
Nelson's bits and pieces come to value transience,
the inevitability of change, even disintegration.
Hers is not a narrative of fixity, stability, surety.
It queerly romances instability. In a long-term
relationship with a trans man, Nelson is adept
at rendering her queer life, loves, and choices as
the product of both experience and theorizing,
her interests in art and critical theory becoming
more than intellectual play but rather modes of
being that are then themselves transformed as
she queerly chooses, queerly loves, queerly lives.
And even when she decides to bear her own
child, his birth nearly dissolves her: "The feeling
has its ontological merits, but it is not really a
good feeling. . . . To let the baby out, you have to
be willing to go to pieces" (134).[3] If anything, what
Nelson seems to value in transience, in the great
uncertainty of it all, is persistence. In choosing
to have a child, she radically de-emphasizes
a heteronormative imperative to reproduce
and rather places emphasis on the necessity of

---

3   Maggie Nelson, *The Argonauts* (Minneapolis: Graywolf Press,
2015).

continuing to choose in the face of transience.
Addressing her child, she says,

> *I want you to know, you were thought of as*
> *possible—never as certain, but always as possible—not*
> *in any single moment, but over many months, even*
> *years, of trying, of waiting, of calling—when, in a*
> *love sometimes sure of itself, sometimes shaken by*
> *bewilderment and change, but always committed*
> *to the charge of ever-deepening understanding—two*
> *human animals, one of whom is blessedly neither*
> *male nor female, the other of whom is female [more*
> *or less], doggedly, wildly wanted you to be.* (142;
> italics in original)

Laced through this declaration, an address to the
futurity represented by the child, weave multiple
moments of radical transience, or the radicality
offered by an awareness and embrace of the
transient. The child is only ever a possibility,
never a certainty, something that can be wanted,
called, and waited for, but whose arrival is never
guaranteed. Similarly, the love claimed to bring
the child into Nelson's family is itself in flux, at
times sure and at others shaken by change. The
primary response to transience is to persist, to
commit oneself to a course of action, a "charge," to
a desire for "ever-deepening understanding"–but
this understanding can be based only on a self–

imposed "charge," a word so close to "change" but also containing within it a trajectory of movement, a thrusting forward, amidst a primary instability.

Again, though, a child. I will not have a child. This book will not birth such an offspring. But from Manguso and Nelson I take the fracturing of text as a kind of grappling with a shifted experience of time. And what I appreciate in Nelson is the perverse valuing of the transient, an embrace of impermanence. I needed that in the immediate aftermath of my stroke. I need it now.

But I also needed even *queerer* feelings. I found myself thinking beyond Manguso's and Nelson's formal approaches to the even more particularly queer nature of how I understood my stroke, of how I had been invited by a homophobic culture to think and feel my body. A pressure that the queer ill contend with is feeling at fault for their condition, of having somehow chosen illness as punishment for their queerness, however subconsciously. Before she wrote about *AIDS and Its Metaphors*, Susan Sontag was already on the trail of the connection between illness and feelings of responsibility in *Illness as Metaphor*. Even though she never discusses queerness in that book, Sontag knew, queer as she was, that "there is a peculiarly modern predilection for psychological explanations of disease, as of

everything else" (709)[4] and, moreover, that "illness
is interpreted as, basically, a psychological event,
and people are encouraged to believe that they
get sick because they (unconsciously) want
to, and that they can cure themselves by the
mobilization of will, that they can choose not to
die of the disease" (710). Sontag was writing in
1978 about the legacies of tuberculosis and the
ravages of cancer, and specifically about the belief
that the repression of feeling causes cancer. But
I read her analyses as articulating a deep truth
about how queer people are encouraged by this
culture to understand any illness they suffer as
essentially self–inflicted, a somatic sign of the
toxicity of queerness itself.

In this guise, the poignant and devastating
beauty of AIDS memoirs became an even more
powerful guide for me. The rich traditions that
have emerged as queer writers have resisted
pathologizing narratives of HIV and AIDS, for
instance, combine both a critique of structures
that stigmatize their illness while also forwarding
a pursuit of pleasure, their ongoing desire for
delight in bodily experience. Even though it is
not about HIV, *Stroke Book* owes much to the work
of queer activists and authors who have written

---

4   Susan Sontag, *Later Essays* (New York: Library of America,
2017).

about the experience of AIDS. Eric Michaels's
Unbecoming: An AIDS Diary taught me about paying
attention to the granular experience of living
with illness, of being in the shadow of death.
David Wojnarowicz's *Close to the Knives: A Memoir of
Disintegration* reminded me of the power of anger
to animate both critique of an unjust world and
a commitment to experiencing as fully as one
can stand it the exigencies and traumas and even
periodic glories of a body coming apart. Perhaps
most importantly, Hervé Guibert showed me in
his fragmented late works, written before his
death from AIDS in 1991, how a queer sensibility
could be both angered by impending death but
also take delight in textual experimentation,
the rough stitching together of fragments of
experience, of desires, of pains, of possibilities
that not only represent but enact a fractured
sense of time, a queer faith in the creative,
an owning of disintegration. I am thinking in
particular here of *To the Friend Who Did Not Save My
Life* and *Cytomegalovirus: A Hospitalization Diary*, both
of which track the dailiness of illness without
sacrificing larger critiques of structures that make
illness worse than it need be.

One particular moment still sticks with me,
from Guibert's *To the Friend Who Did Not Save My
Life*. Critics and commentators are often drawn
in their readings of this book again and again

to its depiction of the last days and death of
Michel Foucault (in the character Muzil) and then
to the narrator's grappling with a friend who
promises access to a potential vaccine but fails
to provide the longed-for medicine. These are,
surely, important narratives. But I keep thinking
of chapter 48, a strange interlude right after the
death of Muzil, in which the narrator recounts
surprising a friend, a priest also dying of AIDS,
with the sight of another friend, a young poet,
casually lying around naked. The priest, a lover
of the young, is naturally delighted: "He was
transported, both mortified and warmed by his
delighted astonishment, ready to fall down on
his knees" (138).[5] The prank assumes its force in
the insistent pursuit of pleasure and forms one
of several such moments throughout Guibert's
work in which the author's writing works against
the pathologization of queer desire, even as
he acknowledges the difficulties of illness, the
injustice of stigma, the pain of being consumed
from the inside out.

Ultimately, though, with consumption comes
the loss of time. Always time, there and then
not. Perhaps what I respond to most in Guibert's
writing is just the extremity of his output, the

---

5   Hervé Guibert, *To the Friend Who Did Not Save My Life*, trans.
Linda Coverdale (South Pasadena, CA: Semiotext(e), 2020).

feverish production, the quite literally *fevered* production, something beyond an urge and approaching more of a demand to record, document, but moreover possibly to transform, to transport, to transubstantiate.

I do not have AIDS. And, as stated, I will not have children. But I reference these works to situate my little book in a larger queer tradition of writing, first, about the body, and then again, about the body unbecoming, and then yet further, about the body ongoing, even in the shadow of death. The pleasure in our unbecoming, which may be the necessary precursor to embracing queerly all of the pleasures of constantly becoming, finds rich expression in the work of younger queer and crip theorists, such as Sami Schalk. In *Bodyminds Reimagined: (Dis)ability, Race, and Gender in Black Women's Speculative Fiction*, Schalk speaks powerfully to ongoing conversations between queer and crip theorists about the ways in which queer stories continue to expose how normative assumptions and pressures on the "healthy" body can be met with counternarratives, with alternative ways of understanding what bodies are for, of what they are capable, of how we can live with and through them, and of how we can reimagine agency over them. Using the work of black women writers, such as science fiction author Octavia Butler,

Schalk shows us the necessity of "understanding disability as a complex experience" and how that "means remaining attentive to positive, negative, and ambivalent aspects of disability (physically, mentally, and socially) as well as the relationship between all three" (24).[6] Schalk's attention to the ravages of racial prejudice on black bodies is vital and necessary; I humbly acknowledge how it has taught me to be more conscious in this book of not just the queer but also the raced nature of my experience of unfolding disability in the aftermath of a health crisis.

Schalk's turn to the speculative is also instructive. For me, the force of a queer approach lies in simultaneous gestures of critique and delight, and even the possibility of *worldbuilding*–and creative worldbuilding through an affirmation of pleasure. In terms of critique, queer resists the pathologization not just of non-heterosexual identities but also of a variety of modes of being, including illness. In this regard, José Esteban Muñoz's desire to "cruise utopia," to cozy up to "the work of not settling for the present, of asking and looking beyond the here

---

6 Sami Schalk, *Bodyminds Reimagined: (Dis)ability, Race, and Gender in Black Women's Speculative Fiction* (Durham, NC: Duke University Press, 2018).

and now" (28)[7] for new intimacies, for queerer
ways of being, feels . . . well, it feels hopeful–and
sexy. And what could feel queerer to me than
being hopeful in the aftermath of an event that
could have killed me, in the acute and embodied
knowledge that I know now how I am likely to
die? What possibilities are opened, what new
intimacies call to me? E. L. McCallum and Mikko
Tuhkanen suggest in *Queer Times, Queer Becomings*
that writing may be the technology that can
(albeit not necessarily) activate the dual critique
and imagination that characterize Muñoz's queer
utopian hermeneutic:

> The temporal complexities between life–as
> a becoming, as a dynamic process of an
> individual's vital and embodied engagement
> with the environment–and language–as
> reading and writing, narrating, or analysis–
> have a power to open up innovative forms
> of intimacy that betoken not only new
> modes of becoming, but new ways of
> affiliation with others and alternative modes
> of transmission. (13)[8]

---

7   José Esteban Muñoz, *Cruising Utopia: The Then and There of Queer Futurity* (New York: New York University Press, 2009).

8   E. L. McCallum and Mikko Tuhkanen, eds., *Queer Times, Queer Becomings* (Albany: State University of New York Press, 2011).

Stroke Book attempts to enact the entangled complexities of critique and imagination, of documenting and analyzing while also holding open a space for dreaming, for pleasure, for intimacy, for the unexpected.

Perhaps what I have ultimately learned from the writing of this book is that there is no experience, no queer experience of health crisis, that is also not an experience of time as *queered*. The blindspot that my stroke left behind has become the fragmentation of my vision that has become the pieces of a narrative–of a self–that has been subject to continual temporal rearrangement, to a backtracking, a questioning, a speculation about my queerness in relation to my stroke, my stroke in relation to my queerness, but also an opening to a future, however now seemingly truncated, that demands, that beckons, that pleads to be felt and lived anew, made up, created, possible.

At least that's what I have come to believe. None of this is easy. But I'm getting ahead of myself. There is so much to say, and only so much time in which to say it.

With that said, a final disclaimer: No time, no queer time, is consistent from person to person, from hour to hour, or even from hour to hour within the phenomenal experience of an individual person. Mine is not yours, just as yours cannot ultimately be mine. But this–*this* is mine, and, perversely, sometimes this isn't even mine, and I invite you to experience what you will of it.

Stroke Book

What does one do with time? Is there a more important question that is as difficult to answer? Of course there is. But this is the difficult question most present in my mind right now, the one about which my life seems to pivot. What do I do with time, especially when I am made aware not just of how little I might have, but of how it might disappear at any moment?

His name is Victor and he took my coffee order this morning. I'm pretty consistent. One petite vanilla bean scone and either a small coffee or a medium Americano. I refuse to use the words "tall" and "grande."

This has been my routine. But his name is a discovery. Victor.

I've been watching him on workday mornings when I come to this Starbucks to get my morning treat, sit with a book, and remain quiet for a few minutes. He doesn't work every morning, so it's always a nice surprise when I see him. This is the first time we've spoken–though, once, he did make my drink and put it on the bar, calling my name. We didn't make eye contact, so I won't count that as an "exchange." But today, when he was taking my order, asking if I wanted *just one* scone and any *room* in my coffee, I risked a joke about *just a little room because it was always filled to the top and that's likely a burn risk.* Small chuckle, diverted eyes. He doesn't know I'm starting to flirt.

Victor. He's Latino, on the shorter side, but not short, a bit stocky. It's his khaki Dickies I position myself to see, his plump butt filling the rough material, stretching it smooth. It's beautiful. Perhaps more beautiful because he's not especially attractive, though hardly ugly. I'm cutting the differences here between

absolutes–pretty, ugly, fat, thin–finding
something absolutely beautiful in the otherwise
unremarkable. But I think Victor might be
remarkable. He might be the most remarkable
part of my day.

I exaggerate. I can't not. But then, as I'm sitting
down with my *Paris Review*, straining my right
eye to see the newly more difficult text, Victor
takes the seat two over from me, no one between
us, pulling out his phone, going on break. No
contact. But I feel him. I look askance, seeing the
khaki–clad legs stretch out a bit, that plump butt
settling into the seat. We won't talk.

I want to. I think I might even try. I'm at
the point, given the week I've had, of saying
something.

Really: I'm not going to fuck this kid. I'm not
even going to masturbate about him. But he's
become a part of my day, even if he doesn't
know it. And taking my order this morning, and
this extra gift of him sitting down so near me–
these feel like *grace*. A beneficence. Something
unexpected. A wrinkle in time.

Like my stroke earlier this week. Unexpected.

There's a story here, obviously, and many ways
to tell it. A little over a month since it's happened
and this is the version I choose to tell right now.
I will have other versions, and the people around
me will have their versions, and the people who
hear secondhand will have their own versions as
well. But this is the story I tell right now.

About a month ago, Mack and I woke up in
our B&B in Colorado, having spent a weekend
looking at real estate and visiting with family and
friends. We'd had a wonderful time, one of those
times that felt like a turning point, a new chapter,
an opening vista, all the cliché things you wonder
if you'll ever feel after having gone through the
clichés of a somewhat darker, less possible time.
(I call that time my forties.) We woke up, ready to
pack our bags and head back to California, but
something, as they say—as I said that morning,
like I was following a script—something was *wrong*.
I couldn't see out of the lower left portion of
my right eye. A curtain had been closed, a veil
descended. A bit of the world grayed out.

I spasmed around the room in my underwear,
fearing a detaching retina. Mack wondered if we
could fly home and have it treated there. I said
no, absolutely not, it has to be seen to *right away*.

(*Seen to*. My failing sight must be *seen* to.)

Hours later, after multiple calls and instructions
from our health insurance provider, we found

ourselves in a medical office outside Denver. Pupil dilation, bright lights, eye-watering scans, and no, my retina was not detaching. Instead, the doctor could see a white spot at the back of my eye, which he surmised was a bit of plaque that had found its way from somewhere else in my body and lodged in a branch artery of my right eye's retina. The plaque was blocking blood flow to that part of the eye, causing what he called an occlusion.

I'd had an "eye stroke."

My blood pressure was also very high. I'd been taking a prescribed diuretic in an attempt to control blood pressure and Zoloft in an attempt to control my stress, but this morning my blood pressure was spiking. *Of course it is. I am going blind*, I said. But the doctor wasn't amused. He sent me immediately to the emergency room of the local hospital.

He was worried that the eye stroke–a bit of plaque blocking an artery–was the beginning of a much more substantial cerebral event: another bit of plaque blocking an artery in my brain.

August 19. A Monday.

That's the day I woke up with partial vision. That's the day I was admitted to the hospital. That's the day on which what we will come to call the "incident" happened. I guess, technically, the "incident" could have happened sometime on August 18, after I'd gone to sleep, but more likely August 19, as I was up late reading the previous night.

Reading.

In the immediate aftermath, all I could think was: *Will I read again, out of that eye, my "good" eye?* The question haunted me for days. Part of me didn't want to know the answer. Part of me didn't want to know the ensuing consequences if I *couldn't* read. My livelihood, English professor, depends upon reading. What happens if I *can't?*

At the time, I couldn't say, but what I *did* know, unequivocally, was that August 19 is a turning point. There is now a clear before and a clearer after. Or, perhaps, less clear in some ways. (I can't seem to resist these little puns.)

August 19.

This is the beginning of this story, but I don't always know what the beginning is. Maybe better to say that I'm choosing to begin this story in this way but that, inevitably, there are other beginnings, possibly infinite beginnings.

Reminding myself of this will come to seem important.

I interrupt this narration to tell you of the immense joy I have in telling you this story. I have to tell you *now* because this joy will not last. It passes. It passes understanding. No, I was not joyful when this was happening to me, though I was not exactly suffering either. More like in limbo. Unmoored. Adrift. (More on this in a bit.)

But in this moment, sitting at this desk, the sunlight behind me, an almond crunching in my mouth, the coffee in my cup getting colder, I don't really care. I am joyful. I'm not sure there's anything else I'd rather be doing. And I am joyful enough to not care that I am lying when I say that. I must be. But at this moment, swallowing bits of masticated almond, I am delighted to be telling you this.

So, back to the hospital (and I'm going to narrate this in the *now*–partly so you can experience it in the *now* and partly because I seem never not to be experiencing this).

Skyrocketing blood pressure, at one point 180/110, and the doctors decide to keep me overnight, running their various tests, CAT scan, bloodwork, ultrasounds, etc. I will be released the following day, the vision in my right eye still partially impaired. But I at least will be cleared to fly back home.

I don't know how to feel throughout this. I'm relieved I'm being seen to, taken care of, tended by Mack, who is so good in an emergency. Friends start texting their concern and love. Mother calls me, worried. I feel comforted.

And then I want to die. I wonder, half hoping, that this is it, this is done, the moment has finally arrived. We can stop now. Whatever this is, it can stop, I can stop.

Karen, one of my oldest friends, who lives in Colorado, drives two hours up to Denver to be with us that morning. She holds my hand. We joke with the neurology resident who comes to see me. The resident thinks we're married. Then Mack comes in, and she's confused. The three of us laugh. Just like old times.

I turn to Karen, still holding my hand. "Too soon. This is just too soon."

I sleep when Karen leaves. I wake up. I throw up, likely from the stress, the relief, the fear. I don't know how to feel about any of this.

A case study.

Patient is a fifty-one year old man in reasonable health. Six feet, 230 pounds, white. Exercises regularly. No history of stroke or heart disease. Some mild blood pressure currently being treated with hydrochlorothiazide, a diuretic designed to help reduce the salt content of his blood and thus reduce blood pressure. Not diabetic. Not particularly high cholesterol. Reports a moderate diet of mostly poultry, vegetables, and some red meat, including turkey and pork.

Patient seems in reasonably good spirits, despite what's happened. Joking with nurses, doctors, and other hospital staff. Mildly inappropriate. Perhaps a good sign.

Patient might begin wondering why this has happened to him, why, given his relatively low risk factors for an eye stroke, this incidence has occurred and what it means for his future.[9]

---

9   I didn't realize until I re-read Hervé Guibert's *To the Friend Who Did Not Save My Life* that Guibert performs a similar kind of narrative accounting at times, stepping to the side, as it were, of his own story to emphasize the different ways one can bear witness to an event, an incident, however personal. Guibert, of course, is documenting his death from AIDS. Linda Coverdale's translation was republished by Semiotext(e) in June 2020.

Patient is a gay man.

(This fact doesn't appear on any of the documentation, but I write it out anyway, as though a part of the case study.)

At first, this will not seem a particularly relevant part of the story. Not one of the various doctors the patient sees seems to care that his partner, the man who is accompanying him, asking questions, staying the night, is in fact a man. Not a woman. A man. So it can likely easily be assumed that the patient is gay. Though no one will ask if he is. It is not deemed relevant. There's at least someone there who can help take care of the patient once he's discharged. The sex of the individual no longer makes any difference.

But perhaps it does, secretly, to someone who is helping the patient, such as a doctor or a nurse or an orderly, someone who harbors inside a homophobic thought or feeling, who internally disapproves but knows that this disapproval is no longer so widely shared that it can be assumed to be part of a communal value system. Too bad, but that's the way some things go. So whoever this might be just keeps quiet. They will not readily tip their hand. Not right now. Perhaps in the past, but not now.

But positively, over and beyond these thoughts of bias and secret discrimination, the patient's sexuality doesn't seem important. Other questions are asked. Age. Health. Exercise regimen. Diet. Medications. Medical history. Family history. Married? Yes, but the sex or gender of the spouse doesn't matter. Not explicitly.

Unless it does, *the patient begins to think.* Not immediately, but maybe it will.

And in fact, we speak too soon. Evening comes and the nursing staff changes. The large hunky white nurse, Matt, is rotating off duty, and another one, a chunky white woman, comes in to introduce herself. She updates the white board with her information. She notices that Mack's name is not listed on the board. She asks his name and goes to write it on the board, marking down the word "partner" to describe his relationship to the patient.

"No, I'm his husband."

"Okay, partner," she repeats.

"No. Husband," Mack insists.

She pauses. Thoughts twist her face. "Ok, yes. I'm going to write 'husband!'"

Mack doesn't thank her. He can't wait for her to get out. He's wondering if she didn't want to pay attention to him because he's Latino, part Native Mexican. Whites don't always have to listen to "those people." Perhaps she sees me and thinks, *OK, I'll do this for the white guy*. We'll never know.

The patient watches all of this and doesn't seem to respond. He's already encountered enough shock today. This bit of haggling is just a bit too much, the icing on the cake that tips you into a diabetic coma. Best for him to ignore it, otherwise it will lodge in his mind, expanding, ballooning, inflicting even further damage that the tiny globule of cholesterol couldn't inflict because it got stopped in the patient's eye.

But he'll feel bad about this later. He'll feel he should've spoken up. He'll feel, as the white man in the room, that he should've said something.

The patient is a gay man. A white gay man. It matters. It all always matters.

I drift into the third person so easily when writing this case study. I am talking about myself. This is not only deflection. But it is that, surely.[10]

---

10   Again, Guibert trod here before me.

We have been here before, and I can switch back
to the first person to tell this story because, while
it took place in another clinical situation, I wasn't
the object of medical scrutiny.

Years ago, well over a decade, in another town,
in the Midwest, another part of our lives, Mack
calls from work, in severe abdominal pain. I rush
to pick him up, take him to the emergency room
where we wait for hours while the doctors run
their tests, poking and palpitating his stomach.

Hours into this scene, the diagnosis crystalizes:
appendicitis. Mack needs emergency surgery. But
it should be fairly routine, nothing much to see
here. Hour and a half or so.

Hours later, I'm in the surgery waiting room.
An hour and a half goes by. Two hours. Two and
a half hours. Nearly three. It's midnight. I get up
and go ask the nurse on duty, a white woman,
what's going on.

"And who are *you*?"

I wish I could describe to you the tone of this
question, laced with contempt, incredulity. *Who
are you to be asking about this patient?*

Perhaps I'm just tired. Perhaps I'm stressed. A
little traumatized from this whole day of medical
emergency. But I realize immediately that I have
no rights here. This is well before gay marriage.
This is well before people in this part of the

country started to give a shit, or at least hide the fact that they don't.

"And who are you?"

"Who am I?" I lean close to her, not minding one bit that the gesture is just a little threatening.

"I'm the only person here asking."

A beat, and then she tells me what I need to know. Perhaps because I'm white. I wonder if she would've been so cooperative if I were, say, Latino, Native Mexican. But no, she tells me. *Everything will be fine.*

The patient is a white gay man. It mattered then. Absolutely.

What also matters is that, back in Colorado,
in between tests while we are waiting in the
emergency room, hours clicking by, wondering
what the hell is going on, only knowing that
something is wrong, I'm rolled into a cubbyhole
where a polite young white woman asks
about insurance. She wants to know, as the
representative of the hospital, which will want to
know, *who will pay for all of this*. And this, before we
really know what's wrong with me.

Who will pay for this?

We sign forms. Yes, we will pay. Yes, there's
insurance. Yes, we will pay if the insurance
doesn't pay.

I'm aware enough in the moment, despite the
shock of the situation, to register that this can't
be good for my blood pressure. This can't be
good. None of this can be good. That, right in the
middle of an emergency, one that doctors haven't
diagnosed entirely but that is nonetheless being
addressed as a life–threatening event, I'm being
asked: *Who will pay for this? Will you assume complete
financial liability?*

What if I'd said *no*? What if I'd said I *can't*?

I'd been here before, curiously enough in Colorado, in a much earlier part of my life. My first marriage, and my wife and I had been in a car accident. We were both in our twenties. Not our fault. A woman ran a red light, plowed into our car, pushed us into an oncoming car. My wife was taken from the scene unconscious. I couldn't move my left arm, my collarbone having been broken by the seatbelt. That's how intense the force of the crash was.

I remember being put in the ambulance, my wife strapped down to a stretcher. She gains enough consciousness to start crying. I'm directed to a seat, and the paramedic starts yelling at me to put my seatbelt on. But I can't. I can't move my arm.

At the hospital, my injury not deemed life-threatening, I'm rolled into a waiting area with a host of others seeking help. I have blood splattered down the front of my white shirt. I'm not sure where it's from.

Hours pass.

I have no idea what's going on with my wife. No one has come to tell me anything. I still can't move my arm.

Finally, someone approaches and starts to roll me to a cubbyhole. I think, finally, I'm going to get some help, I'm going to find out what's going on.

At this point, I still think I might have caused the accident. I don't know that a woman had run her red light, oddly enough on the way to the hospital because she'd just gotten a call that her son had fallen off his bike and cracked open his skull.

But I won't hear about any of this because the cubbyhole I've been wheeled into is all about finances.

"And how will you pay for this?"

"What?"

"Sir, do you have insurance?"

"What? What the fuck?"

"Sir . . ."

"Can someone *please* tell me what's going on? What happened? What the fuck happened? Where's my wife? Is she ok? Can someone please tell me what the fuck is going on?"

I start crying.

"Sir, I'll get someone to help you, but I need you first to sign these forms about financial liability."

What could I do? I couldn't move my arm. I used my other arm to sign the papers.

For all of this history with hospitals, however limited, I experience a weird comfort in my hospital room. I know that part of me is terribly frightened. I know, cognitively, that I'm in the midst of a traumatic experience. But I'm also strangely comforted.

Doctors, nurses, other specialists come and go, and they are all tending to me. They are all interested in how I'm doing. They are poking and prodding, sure, and the blood draw in the middle of the night is not something particularly welcome. Except, in a way, it is. I'm OK with it. I'm being tended to.

People care. I have signed the forms assuming financial liability.

People care. No matter what happens to me, the doctors, the nurses, the specialists, the hospital—all will be paid.

Why do I marvel at the experience of such care?

Some historical context might be useful here. But I'll keep this short. This past is with me enough already.

I grew up in the Deep South of Louisiana, in New Orleans, which outsiders understand as a let-the-good-times-roll kinda place, but which is still in the Deep South for those of us born and raised there.

I went through puberty in the 1980s, when AIDS seemed god's just punishment for the wicked. And by the time I started having sexual thoughts in the 1980s, I knew that I was very likely wicked. A homosexual. A faggot. Queer.

I believed more than anything, more than in the existence of god himself, that I would likely die of AIDS. Because that's what happens to the wicked. That's what happens to homosexuals.

God himself didn't need to exist for this truth to be inexorable. Everyone said so. My church, my school, my parents, my friends, our neighbors, our community, our president. You see, silence is always consent. Silence is always consent. Ronald Reagan didn't have to talk about AIDS for me to know that he fully approved of the widespread death of homosexuals. And there were many, so very fucking many, who weren't silent at all. They knew, and delighted in saying what they knew: Homosexuals die of AIDS, slowly, painfully, unloved, unwanted, uncared for.

So my psyche was trained from early on: *The world hates you and those like you, so take any care you can get.*

Even this nurse in the hospital, the one who didn't at first want to list Mack as my husband, she's still caring for me. We can overlook her sins, Mack and I. After all, I'm still just a queer. A faggot. A homosexual. And she's choosing to overlook that, or so it seems.

And at least I don't have AIDS.

This is important.

Some of us learn to live with anxiety. I'm not sure I know how to live without it. When most of your life is organized around flight, fight, or freeze–with an emphasis on flight or freeze, because hey, those are less likely to result in you getting your ass kicked–you don't know how to stop feeling anxious, even when you're not being directly threatened.

When, from earliest childhood, the bullies–my church, my school, my parents, my friends, our neighbors, our community, our president–when the bullies hate you, and even those not the bullies but those who say they *love* you really don't approve of you, no, not at all, then you start to freeze inside.

(I might as well shift from the second person to the first. I will have to learn to own this story.

After all, I will have to learn to "take it easy," for my health. I'm not sure what else might shake loose in my body and try to kill me. So I will have to learn to be still, not so anxious all the time.

Perhaps this will be like freezing.)

Not everyone will understand this story. Not everyone should. And I'm actually glad for this. If you were born in a different time and place, perhaps later than I was and more on an East or West Coast, then you're not likely to know quite the anxiety that has become my constant companion, my most trusted friend. Because I know he'll never desert me.

And I'm glad for you. Truly. I hope this is you.

I heard a young queer writer, actor, and filmmaker recently talk about his coming out. He grew up in Jackson, Mississippi, so I initially thought that his story might be like mine. But no, he's so much younger. Times have changed, even in Jackson, Mississippi. Sure, not *totally*. His parents weren't happy. They sent him to a therapist. But not a reparative therapist, mind you; a legit therapist to help him cope with being gay.

I'm glad about this, even as I resent it just a little bit. Not that he got help. Not that he's okay. But that, just a couple of decades earlier, my story seems so different, so fucking different.

Different times, different places. Stories shape us, but always in space and time, which shape the stories.

I cannot give you my space and time. I would not wish it on you. But I will tell you about it. I hope you won't *fully* understand it, not in your bones, in your quaking bones, where it counts. But I still need to tell you about it.

Growing up in the Deep South, in the 1980s.
Reagan's America. The height of AIDS in America.
The fear of dying from being homosexual. The
fear of eternal damnation.

I say it again. I repeat myself. This is the history
that never leaves me. These are the times and
the places that are never far from me. I would
say, this is the context that conditions my vision.
These are the bits and pieces of my life that are
rarely out of my sight.

They are also the bits and pieces that can
become dislodged at times, and want to kill me.
They are there even when I don't see them, even
when they look like a blindspot.

What can one see? What can one ever really see?

There is now a point, right below my center of vision, what they call a blindspot. It looks like a mangled piece of gray pizza. Dark gray when I first wake up, almost translucent in bright sunlight. So it has a life of its own, a changeableness throughout the day. It's living inside me, inside my eye, this dying of the light.

In time, the doctors say, I'll notice it less. My brain will adapt. And they will be right. But for now, gray. I see it all the time, even when my eyes are closed.

If it were just a bit higher, I would likely not be able to read out of that eye, my good eye, the eye through which I have seen most of the world, especially books and computer screens–which are, which have been, in some ways, most of my world for most of my life.

What I have feared is losing the "most" of my world.

I wait three days after coming home from the hospital to pick up a book and see if I can read. I lie in bed, like I always do before going to sleep, and reach for the book I'd been reading the night before the "incident," take a deep breath, slowly open it, and read a few lines.

I start to cry.

I can read, at least for now. My world isn't totally blown to shit. At least for now.

I ask my doctor for Xanax. I'd had it before, doled out by a psychiatrist to help with anxiety, but I hadn't had any for a couple of years. I thought it might help with my periodic feelings of being overwhelmed. I wanted something to help me sleep.

She really didn't want to give me any, and the pharmacy attached to my doctor's office made me sign forms as though I were asking for heroin. *It's just fucking Xanax*, I thought. *I know you don't want me to pop them like candy. But help me out here, fucking help me out.*

I wake up in the middle of the night, every night, wondering if I'm going to lose the rest of my vision. I don't want to wake up and have that be the first thing on my mind. Every night. I'd rather sleep through that, please.

Please.

She gives me twenty pills.

I don't take any right away. Not at first. I will, but later.

Just four days after the incident, in an effort to get back to normal, I'm back at work, talking to a large room of parents whose kids are about to start college. I'm to give them words of wisdom to ease their fears of separation.

"You're kids are in good hands. We've got this. *They've* got this. They are ready, even if you aren't.

"You'll be fine."

I offer my platitudes, which seem particularly moving to me this time. I'm on point. I'm sharp. I'm warm and welcoming, reassuring. I've got this.

Applause and then I go to step off the stage, approaching a set of short steps and realize that I don't know how to get down. I can't see out of the periphery of my good eye. I'm so used to looking straight ahead when I walk that I realize I can't see the stairs *unless I look directly at them.*

I don't think anyone sees me falter, or hesitate. It's important to me in that moment that they don't see me hesitate.

I make my way down the stairs and wonder, *what next?*

I realize in a flash that I am unbecoming, yes, but just a piece for now.

Like something has fallen off, lost.[11]

---

11   I take the word "unbecoming" from Eric Michaels's extraordinary diary of his last days, dying from AIDS: *Unbecoming* (Durham, NC: Duke University Press, 1997).

It is hard to talk about what a day is like when you're learning to see again. Everything seems new. Someone goes to shake my hand and I have to adjust my own angle of approach or I will just miss his hand by inches.

I go to work and tilt my head so that I can better see the screen.

I have polite and concerned conversations with co-workers who want to know how I'm doing. But only so much. It's all a bit too much, and I readily agree: not fun to encounter oneself so mortal, not polite to remind each other how fragile our sight is, our lives are.

I start looking carefully at the packages of food I buy. *Any cholesterol in this?* I ask my phone, *does wine have cholesterol?* I'm relieved the answer is no.

I sit with a cup of coffee and feel grateful to be here. I watch the young people in the coffee shop flicker by, laughing, talking loudly. I'm grateful they are here.

I sit with a glass of wine in the evening. I put it down and pick up my phone. My other hand goes for the glass of wine to take another sip, and I miss it by inches. I misjudge the distance. I'm off *by inches.*

I spend my days counting those inches, learning to recalibrate how I reach out to the world around me.

There are many visits to various doctors. Everyone wants a piece of this, it seems. But not all pieces are the same.

The ophthalmologist dilates, scans, peers, fascinated by the plaque he can see, the retinal swelling that he says should subside, the possibility of something called neo–vascularization, as the retina attempts to create alternative blood routes to feed the oxygen–deprived part of my eye. Contrary to what I imagine, this would be a bad thing, creating more complications. But it can be fixed. I think he's eager to have something to fix, because the plaque is going nowhere. It can't be fixed.

I hear how lucky I am that it's not worse.

And then the neurologist, who clearly thinks I'm wasting her time. She's nice about it, though. Smiles. Goes through the motions, has me squeeze her fingers, resist her hands pushing down on my legs, etc., etc. I have done this before, many times already, with other doctors, first in the hospital, then later. Nothing to see here. (Oops, too soon.) That is, nothing amiss neurologically, so the visit to her is just pro forma, a box that must be clicked, a check mark made.

Come back when something really goes wrong, in your brain.

I am definitely slower.

The new medications, one to control cholesterol, one to lower my blood pressure more aggressively, take an immediate toll. I start telling people that I feel someone has taken the control knob on my life and *turned it way down.*

I am slower, which makes everything around me seem slower.

I'm glad it's still the summer and the work in my office is relatively relaxed. We plod along on campus. Nothing seems urgent. Just busy enough to be distracting.

But slower.

Honestly, I'm not that concerned. For someone who has been anxious his entire life, I'm actually glad to be a bit *slowed down.* For a chunk of the day, it doesn't feel like a problem. But then, I'm wrong. There *is* something inside that wants it to be a problem, that wonders why I'm so slow, so tired, wanting to take naps in the middle of the day when I never ever wanted to do so before.

But then again, I think I'm mostly good with it. I go with it. After all, now, worrying feels deadly. Anxiety might trigger another "incident," loosen something else that could kill me. So I'm fine, for now, with being slower.

But for how long?

The week after we get back, I decided to train up to Los Angeles for the day, about an hour's ride north. I ostensibly go to visit a friend, with whom I'm working on a book. What I really want to do is to see if I can do it.

To *see.*

And I do it. It's not bad. Mack drops me off at the train station, and I can navigate the train to Union Station (I'm just sitting on the train after all), and at Union Station I transfer to the Red Line, the subway to Hollywood.

That's where things get . . . interesting. So many people. So many fucking people. I'm overwhelmed by the crowd. I go slowly, afraid I'll run into someone, afraid I won't see them.

I immediately think that I'm glad I'm not in New York, like earlier this year, where it's so easy to get lost, to be pushed and jostled, to be crowded, to feel crowded out of your self as you switch from one subway to another. Here, I at least know where I'm going, having made this trek so many times in the past.

But I go slowly. I have to pay attention. All I can think of is how to hold on to myself.

What was before like?

Before.

Before, that is, August 19, before the "incident."
(I think to myself, why am I still putting that in
quotation marks, the quote–incident–unquote,
as though it weren't a completely real thing,
something that maybe *could* have happened,
but didn't, or something already becoming
mythic in ways that cast doubt on the verifiable
materiality of the occurrence? But I see, everyday,
the reminder of the incident, a reminder that is
a hole, a lacuna, a gap, a missing part of what I
once had in my right eye.)

Before is everything that is now not there.[12]

---

12   It's so interesting reading these lines long after I first
wrote them, reading them in 2020, in the midst of the COVID
pandemic, when I use the word "before" to describe not just
before my incident but now before the larger incident, the
pandemic, the lockdowns, the rising death toll, and to feel
myself newly vulnerable, in a high–risk category. I footnote
this because it seems ancillary to the main story I'm telling,
but then I think, is it? Is it ancillary? Isn't it too *the* story?
There is before, and then not before. What we narrate is all
about *scale.*

I tell my doctor that I feel tired, that the new blood pressure medicine is making me slower. It's taken a good twenty points off my pulse.

I think to myself: *I'm not fighting, or taking flight, or even freezing anymore. I'm just meandering. Sauntering.*

She nods and smiles, pats my hand and says, "That's what health feels like."

I lean in and say, "Fuck your health. I don't like it." I'm really just joking, I think. Just a little joke, talking about this change that's come over me.

Fortunately she laughs. She's being patient with me because I've had a "trauma." Indeed, she reminds me that one of the reasons I likely feel tired, or slow, is that I've had a "trauma." I'll recover, she assures me.

Can she? Can she assure me? Fortunately, I'm slow enough not to worry about being reassured.

And then, at other times, maybe ironically because I feel so much slower, I feel my animal self. Something embodied. Something *raw*. I'm taking the time to feel it, not rushing past it. The animal.

I don't know how else to describe it.

I'll be sitting somewhere, and my flesh starts to quiver, pulses. I feel my pulse, gently drumming in my neck, starting to move my whole body in a slow rhythm.

I feel myself throb. I feel animal.

And then, in the middle of the night, I wake up, wondering if I can still see. But immediately notice that I'm fully erect. I'm in my fifties. I'm rarely fully erect in the middle of the night.

The animal is still inside me, throbbing, asking to be noticed, wanting to be noticed. Waiting.

But for what?

The night before the "incident" I was reading Wayne Hoffman's novel *Hard*. Lovely book, about being young and gay in the '90s in New York. The narrator is a college student, a journalist, a writer, an AIDS activist. In the '90s in New York. An exciting time, a thrilling if painful time. A time of activism, community building, political struggle, death, life in the midst of death, and vice versa. Queers *alive*, even in the midst of death.[13]

Queers *hard*.

Time and place again, always time and place. This character's life is so different, this fictional life, than the one I've had.

I remember my first AIDS test, very early '90s, in Baton Rouge, LA, the white nurse drawing the blood and shaking her head. What a shame. What a pity. That I would even *want* to have this test.

A quarter century later that nurse is still with me. She's telling me, *See? You read this filth, you sickening homosexual? See what happens? Use what's left of your sight to see how sick you are.*

---

13   Wayne Hoffman's *Hard* is the prequel to *An Older Man*, and both are gay romances about a portly gay bear who loves to suck cock. *Hard*, originally published in 2006, was reissued by Bear Bones Books in 2015. Please support indie queer publishing.

I know she's wrong. Everything I know as an intelligent and educated human being knows that she's wrong.

I still haven't finished reading Wayne Hoffman's *Hard*.[14]

---

14 I eventually did finishing reading it, if you're curious.

If thy eye offend thee, pluck it out.[15]

But whose voice is this, telling me that it offends me? And who is offended? And why should I care? Why should I care if they are offended? Why should I care if they are offended when I have spent much of my life convincing myself that I have no good reason myself to be offended?

Or maybe, is my eye somehow offended on my behalf? On behalf of him who has otherwise convinced himself that he is not offended?

Does my eye know better?

And whose voice is this now? Who is talking? What speaks in me, through me, for me?

Who are you?

---

15 You can find the chapter and verse in a Bible of your choice. I don't feel like helping you.

Maia Dolphin-Krute writes about her own chronic illness in *Visceral: Essays on Illness Not as Metaphor*. She describes how memoirs of illness are often, though not always, stories of a "single event" followed by a "heroic struggle, or journey." She wants to theorize about this narrative proclivity, tell its meta-story, blending her own life writing with theory.

But then she breaks. There's always a body. There's never *not* a body. And how much, she asks, "How much theory can a body take?"[16]

And another question: How much heroic struggle can a body take?

And more, in my less heroic, less theorized moments: What is my body telling me? What does my eye want to tell me?

---

16   Maia's wonderful book was published by punctum (small "p" intentional) in October of 2017.

"What was the thread that held together the scattered beads of experience if not the pressure of interpretation?"[17]

---

17 The narrator of Edward St. Aubyn's *Some Hope* asks this. *Some Hope* is part of the Patrick Melrose novels about a man dealing with the aftermath of severe childhood sexual abuse at the hands of his father.

I want to tell a different story right now.
Something about a boy. Something about the
boy I saw early this morning, a young man,
walking across a bridge away from the coffee
shop I'd just left. A boy in his khaki shorts,
something about a pair of khaki shorts that
always draws my attention, my eye, my formerly
good eye, on constant alert for the khaki-clad
bottom, the fleshy-colored material cupping a
boy's behind.

I walk behind him a little bit, stare fixed on
his ass, noting the creasing of cloth in his crack.
I theorize: He must be wearing boxers for there
to be that much bunching in his crack. Briefs
or boxer briefs would sculpt his butt a bit more
carefully, following the curvy contours of his
flesh, allowing the khaki shorts to bend with his
behind as it pumps out his strides.

I continue to stare, theorizing.

I want to spend part of every day in such
meditations, studying the ass cracks of young
men as they pass me by, the folds of material
moving around a sphincter awaiting, perhaps
guarded, perhaps welcoming, perhaps totally
oblivious, but pulsing still, pumping, moving
itself. This boy may not know yet what he can do
with his ass, what his ass is already doing, what

possibilities it calls forth. Or he may know all too well.[18]

The world in an ass, waiting, drawing my eye to everything.

---

18   For more on ass watching, check out my *Creep: A Life, a Theory, an Apology*, published by punctum books in late 2017. The third section, "An Apology," will be particularly revelatory. Or creepy.

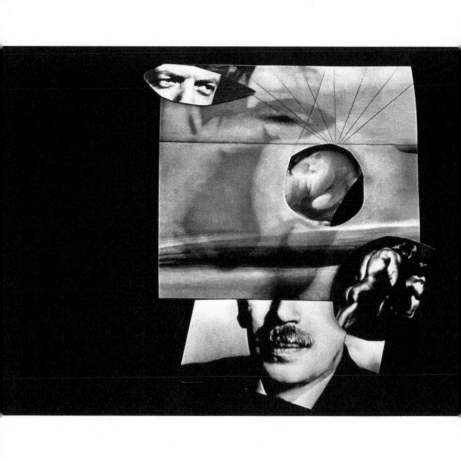

After returning home from Colorado, the hospital, "the incident," I'll figure out how to feel about what has happened. Or at least I will start the process of trying to figure out how and what to feel. That's what I keep telling myself.

I note the figuring here. A calculation.

We tend to think of our feelings as the most natural part of who and what we are. But are they? They are constantly being manipulated by the worlds we inhabit, and we too are constantly manipulating them—chemically, situationally, aesthetically. Through the people we choose to hang around. Through the events we choose to participate in. Through the problems we cultivate with love, assiduously, holding on to our pains and slights, not just the promises and joys, imagined or otherwise.

I have become well aware of how and what I cultivate in myself. The habitual turn to worry unless I catch myself. The familiarity of resentment. The sadly infrequent embrace of unfettered joy.

There seems always to be a fettering. A calculation.

Surely none of this, this cultivation, is without effort, even if just the effort to see more clearly what we are doing, what we are doing to ourselves—or to refuse to see.

And yes, sometimes we fail to see; we are overwhelmed. We succumb.

Even this abstraction here, this abstraction is a form of feeling, a distancing of feeling that is still feeling, a relationship to feeling. Even this abstraction *about* feeling is something I cultivate because I don't know how to feel about what has happened, about "the incident."

I don't know how to feel right now.

What actually happened? I ask myself this
question many, many times.

I had gone to bed the night before after a
weekend of rich food, visits with friends and family,
a drive up and down the state of Colorado on I–25.
During the night, a piece of cholesterol broke off,
likely from one of my carotid arteries, one leading
away from my heart and toward my head, and
lodged in a branch artery of my right eye.

Yes, we'd eaten richly, but no, I wasn't
otherwise at great risk for such a stroke. Yes, I
was already being treated for mild high blood
pressure, but for some reason my blood pressure
was spiking, possibly all weekend long. The
elevated pressure–exacerbated by the altitude–
worked something loose.

I'd also taken the night before an Imitrex,
which had been prescribed to help treat my
periodic migraines. What no one told me was that
Imitrex can also increase your blood pressure.
So, a confluence of factors likely created a unique
situation.

I am unique. Perhaps even an outlier.
Something rare. Queer.

But what actually happened? I can only
theorize. But such theories guide my experience
of the aftermath, of how I attempt to shape a
life in the aftermath of this unique, potentially
anomalous incident. This queer incident.

A digression.

What feels *queer* about this? And then, what feels queer about *time*?

The primal question: How did you get this way, partially blinded? Echoing the other primary question of my life: How did you get to be *queer*?

Your attempt to answer such questions–this imperative to account for yourself, to justify your being–assumes a temporal form, the origin and etiology taking shape as a series of moments in which you might be able to identify the wrong turn, the unfortunate bend in the road, even if such is only a genetic twist of fate.

You must give an accounting of yourself.[19]

You must account for how you *went wrong*.

---

19 Thinking here, of course, of Judith Butler's *Giving an Account of Oneself* (New York: Fordham University Press, 2005), which Google curiously identifies as a "self-help book."

Perhaps the anomalous nature of the experience prompts the doctor to treat me with extra care when I return home and see her. Previously she'd always seemed rushed, busy, even impatient. *Many people to see today, many people.* But now I suspect she wonders what she missed, what she might have done wrong, what she might have done differently.

She's just experienced a death in her family, she tells me.

So she sits with us, almost commiserating, almost as though what has happened to me has also happened to her.

I won't lie: I'm tempted to accuse. *What did you miss? Why didn't you treat my high blood pressure more aggressively? Why didn't you warn me about the Imitrex? Did you just assume that, as a queer man without children (so unlike you, married white gal with children), that my life was oh so much simpler than yours, that it was all fun and games, as long as I practice safe sex? What are your blindspots, doctor?*

But, despite myself, my forming anger deforms into sympathy. I'm infected with her empathy. I avoid resentment, which will only increase anxiety, working something else loose from the past that could harm my future. I have to start thinking of the aftermath, of the right now. It's what I have left.

I have been dwelling at the beginning of this story, but, like I've said, I don't always know what the beginning is.

So, to start again.

I might begin with the rich food we'd had all weekend long, the green chili–covered burger I'd had the previous night, the green chili–slathered tortellini at the new Italian place in town the night before, the bottles of wine, the rich egg-heavy breakfasts at the B&B.

We didn't eat like this all the time. We had, in fact, over the last several years become far more conscious of our dietary consumption. Maybe not enough, but *working on it*, as they say, as we ourselves said. But this weekend we partied. We played. We indulged. A turning point. Thinking of buying a second home, an investment property in a state we loved. Thinking of retirement. Thinking of end points, but not too soon. Kicking the ball down the road a bit. But preparing, seeing the ball, getting ready to make our play.

I could go back further to a time before we were working on it. Even before Mack and I were together. A young adulthood, struggling with coming out, drinking too much, unmindful of diet, not caring what I put in my body, or rather caring mostly that I numb myself by seeking out certain kinds of foods, sugars, carbs, alcohols.

Self–medicating as they say. As I myself said at the time: *I'm self-medicating.*

I so desperately did not want to be gay. 1980s, south Louisiana, conservative Christian upbringing, Catholic schooling. Next to nothing in my life wanted me to be alive. Audre Lorde puts it this way: "We were never meant to survive."[20]

I learned the lesson well. I tried to kill myself, slowly, however slowly but also assuredly, with food, with junk food, with poisonous food all too readily available for a poor kid in college, surviving term to term on grants and scholarships doled out at the last minute. Some weekends I could only afford Vienna sausages on white bread with a little mustard for taste. These days we call this kind of experience "food insecurity." Food was on a long list of things about which I was insecure.

I was most insecure, traumatizingly insecure, about the state of my immortal soul. I was damned already for wanting that boy in my philosophy class, the writer for the school newspaper, a bit stocky, his greasy brown hair swooping over one eye. I loved that he completely ignored me, likely disdainful if not even contemptuous of my interest, my longing

---

20   This is from her amazing poem "Litany for Survival."

gazes. I fed on his disdain. I ate my sausages on white bread and, when I could, drank something called jet fuel at the local bar, a high-alcohol cocktail that looked like Windex.

It made me feel better. It made me feel *less*.

I'm tempted to start my story here, a time when, so young, twenties, I was already weakening the walls of my arteries and veins, feeding on the foods that would slowly start to clog them, eating my pain, eating the pain given to me by others.

I would eventually know better.

But what lives on inside us? How many things live on inside us, even when we think we have moved on, even when we think we know better?

I live under a death sentence, never knowing
when another little bit of cholesterol will
pop loose and lodge in my brain, cutting off
circulation to some vital part of my body
keeping me alive. A death sentence, with no
known execution date. Just the inevitability, an
inevitability that could be now, or later, or much
later, or sooner.

I don't know.

But isn't that much like living a queer life?
Even in an age of increased tolerance, at least
in some parts of the world? It's also an age of
increased *intolerance* in other parts.

I still walk down the street and wonder: *What
harm does that stranger mean me?*

And then I wonder: *What harm does my wondering
mean me?*

I learn later that large parts of the South, a huge swath of the South, has been identified by doctors as the "stroke belt"–an area that, due to obesity, high cholesterol, poor diets, minimal exercise, increased smoking, and substandard health care, is full of people, higher than the national average, susceptible to stroke.[21]

Stroke belt.

21   The Wikipedia page on the "Stroke Belt" is actually pretty decent and sobering for those of us who grew up in that area: https://en.wikipedia.org/wiki/Stroke_Belt.

Pain. There's just never not pain.

I take selfies of the bags under my eyes.

I just started noticing these bags a couple of years ago. Sometimes they are *pronounced*, as we say. Like canyons forming under my eyes. Gashes through puffy skin. They look painful but I feel nothing. I squint to see them better, wrinkles forming around my eyes, only making the overall effect even less aesthetically appealing.

I keep snapping selfies of my eyes, catching different angles, with and without my glasses, seeing how I might mitigate the awfulness.

I hardly ever, as in really never, notice the bags underneath someone else's eyes. But I see mine. I'm getting older.

I never wanted children, but I'm glad that others will go on. Someone will go on.

I'm also glad that I won't be here. Mack and I hope we will die before things get "really bad," whatever "really bad" means. Ecological catastrophe. Political disarray. We just suspect that the shit's about to hit the fan. We'd like to miss the shit.

But I'm glad others will be here—not because I want them to experience the shitty fan hitting but because it *is* oddly comforting to think that others will keep going, keep pushing, keep striving—or keep relaxing, taking it easy, letting come what comes.

I know I'm not sounding very ethical about this right now. The last thing humanity should be doing is taking it easy. We might be taking it easy right out of existence. But I suspect not. And that's the comfort. Others will pick up where we have left off, perhaps correcting what we've tried to do, but still hopefully appreciating our efforts. But even if not, not appreciating that is, still *continuing*, thinking the fight is worthwhile, the fight to survive, perhaps even to thrive.

Comforting. I don't have to do everything. And for once, I feel a bit relieved of my narcissism. I'm anticipating when I won't be here anymore.

I suspect I sound peculiar. I *am* peculiar, or so I flatter myself.

I've always seen things a bit differently, quite literally.

I've long had trouble with my eyes, and have been noticeably cross-eyed my entire life. Up to this point, my right eye, which is nearsighted, has been dominant, which is useful because I read so much, while my left eye (which is farsighted) has been slowly weakening. The ophthalmologist calls this amblyopia. I can still see out of my left eye, but when I switch back and forth from one eye to another, seeing out of that left eye is noticeably a strain. At best, it feels odd, and I default back to my right eye. Even now, with its blindspot, I'm still favoring that right eye.

Years ago, one optometrist, taking photos of my optic nerves, noted that they were neither identical nor symmetrical in appearance, as they apparently are in most people. Instead, he mused, it's as though I have the optic nerves of two different people, my eyes each having seen the world differently for so long.

"I ate my twin in utero," I once calmly told this optometrist. And he just as calmly suggested that "we don't address those kinds of problems here, sir."

Un Chien Andalou by Luis Buñuel famously begins with a woman's eye being slit open. It's not actually a woman's eye, obviously. I think it's a cow's, a dead cow's. But the image is shocking, was intended to be shocking, was intended as an assault on the bourgeoisie. It's an attempt to conjure the un- and perhaps even anti-rational. To frighten, to *shock*.

I think about this image obsessively in the weeks after my incident. Doing so seems perfectly rational: an obsessive consideration of what seems irrational, of the anti-rational, of that which conjures fright, the fear in my particular case of something that shouldn't have happened, that wasn't likely to happen, that did not exist high on the charts of medical probability.

Something *horrifying*. An eye split open.

My sense of the rational has been insulted, damaged, blinded.

Un Chien Andalou, my new companion. I don't know what this means, but I have lost faith in probabilities. I hold now to the possibilities of the irrational.[22]

22   This feels obvious, referencing *Un Chien Andalou* by Luis Buñuel. But you might consider that, having grown up in a pretty conservative and pretty Catholic part of the US, I find watching Buñuel, even now, into my fifties, a bit transgressive. A deep down part of me long ago implanted by my cultural background responds, knee-jerk, to heresy.

I suddenly recall that, at thirty, thirty-one, I was driving down a road, away from our apartment, probably headed to a bookstore one warm summer day, and I turned a corner and was momentarily blinded by the sun. Just a moment, and when the glare passed, I saw the usual spots, but also some small squiggly lines, like little threads suspended in my right eyeball. The glare spots dissipated, but the lines stayed. Not all the time, but especially in brighter light, or if I was looking at something white, I'd see them, a line with a small knot in it.

I thought I was experiencing a detaching retina, having just learned about such a horror from my brother-in-law, who had to have emergency eye surgery.

I immediately booked an appointment with our optometrist, who, after running his various tests, sat back and said: "Sometimes, when we get older, the fluid inside your eye starts to congeal a little, casting a shadow on your retina. These are called floaters."

"I'm thirty-one."

"I know."

Floaters. Harmless, really. Harmless portents of getting older.

Portents of mortality.

Indeed, another way to think of all of this that has happened to me, my "incident," is as part of the problem of getting older and the concomitant betrayals of the body.

So many betrayals of the body . . .

But what body makes you any promises?

Even given my vision's already somewhat attenuated level, I noticed, a couple of years ago, shortly after Trump became president, a marked loss of visual acuity in my left eye, my "bad" eye. Objects were just blurrier. Some straight lines even appeared curved. At first I just shook my head rapidly back and forth, hoping that I could shake loose the magic snow globe of the eyeball into some kind of clarity, letting whatever was amiss settle back into my normal bad vision.

Shake as I might, nothing was improving.

So I made an appointment with one doctor who then, failing to see anything wrong (except the slow, incipient creep of cataracts), referred me to another doctor, who took a variety of pictures, disappeared for a bit, and then came back into the room where I patiently sat in a chair with numerous torture devices extending around me.

"Mr. Alexander, do you take steroids?"

Not the question I was anticipating, so I responded snarkily, as is my habit: "Do I look like I take steroids?"

Ignoring that, he proceeded: "Are you under an undue amount of stress?"

"Are you kidding me? Am I stressed? Besides the trials and tribulations of being an English professor, yes, I'd say I'm stressed. Have you been watching the news? The election? The inauguration? Our worst nightmares are coming true!"

"I suggest yoga. And perhaps some meditation."

". . ."

"You have central serous retinopathy. A bit of fluid has built up behind your retina and it's distorting your vision. It's usually caused by steroid use or an increase in cortisol, a stress hormone. If you're not taking any medically necessary steroids, then stop taking any medically unnecessary steroids. And if you're not taking any steroids at all, then try yoga and come back in a month. Try to manage your stress better."

". . ."

"See you in a month."

I was, as you can see, speechless. Manage my stress? You might as well ask the universe to undo everything it's done. Ever. Since the beginning of the Trump presidency, my Facebook feed had been brimming over with messages of outrage, despair, annoyance, frustration, anger, sadness—you name a dark emotion. We were all stressed.

Living on the California coast, I knew I could very likely find many yoga studios (as the doctor prescribed), but I suspected that I would find relatively few people in them who were going to tell me that everything is going to be okay. Instead, the mantras of the day were all about keeping the faith against the evil empire, taking to the streets, mobilizing our righteous indignation, and then also worrying over what awfulness will hit next. Compounding the problem, we also recognized–again, an important mantra here–that we shouldn't "normalize" the Trump presidency. We were living in extra-ordinary times and they needed to be treated as such. We needed constant vigilance. We needed to remain on high alert.

But confronting the extra-ordinary on a daily basis is, well, stressful. And my body, or at least one part of it, started reacting negatively to that stress. So I left the ophthalmologist's office that day with a real problem. I'd have to learn to manage my stress at a time when such seemed nearly impossible, or potentially go steadily blind in one eye. The mandate was clear: Relax, and *now*–for your own good.

I took some immediate and simple steps. I limited my Facebook trolling. I told my husband, who had led our household's strategy to canvass for Bernie Sanders, that I couldn't wake up in

the morning to the latest news on the atrocities
of the Trump administration, a litany that had
been serving as his motivating matins. I told him
I would listen to periodic reports, which he was
kind enough to summarize, being a die-hard
news junkie, but I needed to wean myself off the
daily terror. I didn't want to wake up to it.

I also started meditating in the morning, for
at least fifteen minutes, something I hadn't done
in years. At first, it felt so strange, seemed even
somewhat transgressive. Not exactly a waste of
time, but a selfish apportionment of energy that
could otherwise be channeled into direct action
to protest the current regime. But it was one that,
at the time, I needed to help preserve my sight.

Turns out, it wasn't enough.[23]

---

23   I wrote a different version of this—or should I say that
this version is different from the one I wrote in my "before"—
for the *Los Angeles Review of Books*, titled "Blinded by Donald
Trump, or, Slowing Down": https://blog.lareviewofbooks.
org/essays/blinded-donald-trump-slowing/. A comparison
between that text and my mining of it here for this diary
remains instructive to me.

There are many things I can write about, as you can see.

Right now, I want to write about other things, about my own sense of agency, about my own power in the world. About my own control.

But I stop. I catch myself. I make myself write about this experience, this "incident" and its aftermath. I'm not exactly afraid that I will forget. More that I'm afraid that the desire to return to some kind of normalcy will overtake my sensations, my thoughts, my memories of what happened. I don't want to lose the texture of how this all felt, how it *feels*.

And I wonder: Am I talking about my eyesight, or the Trump presidency?

The normal numbs. That's perhaps why we like it, why we allow ourselves to be pulled under its warm blanketing everydayness. The normal accrues, casting shadows of consistency, continuity, and then increasingly the possibility of longevity, permanence.

But this is a shadow world. I'm seeing shadows, I keep telling myself.

I finally go to the gym, after being cleared to do so by several physicians. I want to feel normal again. I want to feel my body again. The animal calls.

By this point, it's been a couple of months since I've worked out. I used to lift weights, wanting to improve my chest, my biceps. But not recently, understandably.

I'm still startled when I discover that I can do so much less now.

Just *less*.

I'm weak. I feel weak, weakened. There's no other word, no other word that comes to mind.

Weakened.

There's before, and then after. At the gym, I'm definitely after.

What's the shelf life of gratitude?

I can feel the old resentments creeping up, wanting to take the periodic, fleeting solace of my newfound slowness by surprise. Resentment, paranoia, *I didn't deserve this, I should've been loved instead.* The old anxieties, the old ways of thinking, my favored habits, my old friends.

The world is out to get me. The universe conspires against us. And just because you're paranoid doesn't mean people aren't out to get you.

This last one is almost a joke, but not quite; I take my paranoia, my anxieties seriously, my old friends, my most faithful companions. When you are raised to hate yourself, you find companionship where you can.

My dear friends.

But now I see them a bit more clearly.

A follow-up appointment, and a doctor says something that hits me, a recognition that I haven't had a chance to confront yet: "We can't stop the plaque already in there."

He wasn't talking about the plaque obstructing blood flow in my eye. He's talking about the plaque that's already coating part of my arteries. *That* plaque. Some of it could come loose and kill me.

We're not done yet.

ssessed for a while with searching for
 images, videos, anything that describes
imals, dogs and cats mostly, see.
t does the world look like to them?
e on images of muddied backgrounds,
ots, grayed-out areas, bits and pieces that,
numan eye, would resolve into some kind
y.
nder if I am becoming more animal.

The flows, the paths, the wrong turn, the
devastation.

I write out this sequence and realize that it
implies—it even *asserts*—the activity of agency at
some point. We're flowing along and then make a
choice, perhaps not entirely consciously, but just
enough to open up the question of culpability
when we arrive at the scene of devastation.

I have arrived. I have questions.

One of my dearest friends, someone who has devoted her life to the study of the classical world, characterizes my incident as an act of divine intervention. But for her, the intervention is a *smiting* and, given her deep affinity for the ancient pagans, a smiting without meaning. Not every act of the gods needs to be understandable, or have a human reason.

"It's like the hand of god came down and smote you."

For her, the question is answered. The smiting is sufficient unto itself.

I look for other answers. It's inev wouldn't, except my classically o and perhaps other pagans resign say) to the fateful vicissitudes of life?

I a
art.
ho

I
bli
wit
of c

I

Back to the past, the "before."

I remember calling my mother to talk about my eyes, not about the incident, but about the earlier problem, central serous retinopathy.

At the time, before she moved in with us, we talked nearly daily and while she's not really that old, only seventy-three at the time, I felt the need to connect with her regularly, to know more about her life, to be open to her stories from the past. I worried for a bit that the election might cause a bit of a rift, as she's fairly socially conservative, attending Mass regularly. But she couldn't bring herself to vote for Trump, even if she couldn't bring herself to vote for Clinton either. So pretty good there, not a Trumper, an incipient fascist.

I told her about my eye, and she, like the doctor, wondered what I have to be so stressed about. I allowed myself a bit of a whine and complained about all the horrible stuff Trump was doing, the recent executive orders banning travel from certain countries topping the list at the moment.

Her response came chillingly: "But really, what is he doing *to you*?"

"..."

I composed myself, realizing it isn't very mature of me at nearly fifty to yell at my mother, however much my inner child wants to. I then calmly explained that, for starters, Trump didn't have to be doing anything in particular to me for me to find his policies abhorrent, his values deeply suspect, his humanity in question. While relatively secure for now, I could still feel terribly for the families torn asunder by his travel ban, for instance. Taking it closer to home, I could certainly begin to worry about the kinds of anti-LGBT legislation that a dominantly Republican administration might attempt to pass in the coming years; Pence in particular seemed worrying on that count. So yes, for the moment, I wasn't feeling myself the toxic effects of this administration, but I also wasn't going to suspend either my empathy for others feeling those effects or ignore the very real possibility that the damage could arrive one day at my own doorstep.

My mother and I stopped talking about Trump, and we have generally avoided political discussions since, but I left the conversation scratching my head about how I might continue to cultivate a capacity for empathy, something of a hallmark of liberal and progressive thinking and being in the world. How could I continue to feel for those damaged by Trump, without my anxiety about that damage damaging *me*?

But at other times, oh at those so many other times, a victim of my own stresses, my own anxieties, blinded in part (I feel) by my own incapacity to manage the stress of it all–I just want it to stop. Whatever it is.

Just stop.

I don't want to see anymore.[24]

---

24 See the previous note about the article published in *LARB*.

I close my eyes and see dilating and flashing spots.

These will subside in time, but for now, in the month or two in the aftermath of the incident, I can't help but see them as foreshadows, the oncoming bardos that separate this life from the next.

Patrick Anderson writes of his own sudden
and then chronic illness in *Autobiography of a
Disease*. I like his blending of genres: storytelling,
historiography, ethnography, memoir.

But also, I think, *why hybridity?* Why is this the
seemingly preferred form these days? What do we
hope to see when genres lose their own distinct
forms, blur at the edges, warp beyond immediate
recognition? Is this, as Patrick says, one of the
ways "we make sense of being–ill"? Is this how we
"care"?

There's a theory here. As he puts it, "This
book . . . understands illness not as a patient's
monologue or biography but as a profoundly
social, richly durational, and multiply perspectival
encounter." Multiple perspectives seems to call for
multiple genres. So, hybridity. Yes, I get that, I do.
I've been writing toward hybridity myself.[25]

But why do I also at times just want a
monologue? a simple statement? a concise
rendering?

This is what happened, and this is why.

---

25   Patrick Anderson's *Autobiography of a Disease* is an amazing
book, published by Routledge in 2017. Google oddly calls it a
"reference book." Something is wrong with Google.

Is it dramatic to say this feels like death, the closing of the blinds? The final pulling of the cover over one's head?

My mother asks, "Do you feel like your life is slipping away?"

Then I wake in the middle of the night, hard.

And I can still see, mostly.

Mostly.

As I suggested earlier, I haven't often woken up with an erection for going on four, likely five years. On the extremely rare occasions when I have over the past few years, I've looked down and wondered what's wrong. *What's happening down there? Is something clogged, perhaps?* I've (mostly) accommodated to my middle age, rationally understanding the steady loss of testosterone and subsequent lowering sex drive as less a loss than a reprieve. I have felt, thankfully, less *driven.*

But after my stroke, for several nights in a row now, I've woken up in the middle of the night, fully erect. I can only articulate my surprise as a kind of gratitude. I am thankful. I feel my body asserting itself. I am still here. I am still here. And more, I am vital. Vibrant, even. Blood is flowing, moving, filling my cock. I am ready. I am here.

Let's do this, whatever this is, whatever comes next.

I've just come back from a follow-up
appointment with an ophthalmologist, a retinal
specialist.

It's two months after the "incident." The
specialist dilates my pupils and shines his
klieg lights into my eyes in the darkened room
while Mack attends to his phone in a chair in
the corner. The doctor then reclines my chair
so he can almost crawl on top of me to peer
even more acutely into my eyes. I sit up, seeing
spots, splotches of darkness accompanying my
blindspot. Out of my right eye, the screen on the
far side of the room, the one upon which they
project letters for you to read, appears white. I
squint and look out of my left eye and it's purple.

I go back and forth, squinting one eye closed to
look out of the other, and the screen goes quickly
from white to purple, white to purple

What has he done to my left eye? Why is it
seeing in purple?

I blink furiously, hoping this purpling will go
away. My vision feels bruised. I want to rub it out.
I panic, thinking I should say something. But I
don't want to. I don't want yet something else to
be wrong, especially now with my "good" eye—
which is ironic since this one has always been my
"bad" eye. (Perspective. It's a kick in the ass.)

So I keep my mouth shut, listening to the
ophthalmologist talk about how lucky I am,

how lucky it is that the plaque didn't occlude my central vision, which would have completely blinded me in that eye. I listen to him but only half hear, as I try to blink away the bruise.

It slowly fades, thank god, and I realize that I'm feeling relieved to be hearing about how lucky I am.

Maia Dolphin–Krute tells a joke in her critical memoir about chronic illness: "How do you live with something for a long time? All of the time, I imagine."[26]

I imagine too. But for how long?

---

26   I haven't given you many page numbers, but this quotation is on page 134 of Maia's *Visceral: Essays on Illness Not as Metaphor* (Goleta, CA: punctum books, 2017). Take that, Susan Sontag.

Still thinking about how lucky I am, and I think of AIDS. Weeks into the aftermath, and I think of AIDS. Then I realize I've never not been thinking of AIDS, for thirty years at least. This was the end meant for me, the judgment ordained by a just god.

I was never meant to survive.

I was just wrong about the delivery mechanism for death.

I feel that I know now how I will die. I've been told in advance: *This is how it likely ends. Not AIDS, but a stroke, a catastrophic stroke.*

No guarantees, though. Nothing is guaranteed but that it will come, whatever it is that shakes loose in a body and kills us.

In *The Picture of Dorian Gray*, Lord Henry Wotton, wooing Dorian, tells him, "Nothing can cure the soul but the senses, just as nothing can cure the senses but the soul."[27]

Whatever Wotton's intentions (and they aren't good), I know as a queer man what Wilde-as-Wotton is trying to say. When you are told, from before birth, that what you are is sinful, deranged, and damned, then your soul has already all but died. So, you wager, you need the evidence of the flesh to remake your soul.

Almost everything I've done to remake myself I've done through my eyes. They have allowed me to look at that which I desire, to hold my gaze on it, not to turn away like I'd been taught, like I'd been warned and threatened.

What are you looking at, faggot?

No, I have learned, have forced myself to hold my gaze. The khaki-clad ass in the Starbucks, or walking down the street. Victor, dear Victor at the coffee stand. In this way, I've remade myself.

But for how much longer? I fear their darkness will overtake me yet.

---

27   In a perfect world, when googling *The Picture of Dorian Gray*, Google would identify this extraordinary novel as a "self-help book."

And then I think, wait. Yes, wait, really. *What if your senses are damaged? What then happens to your soul? Aren't all of us, only ever temporarily able-bodied, if that, always on the verge of losing our souls?*

Perhaps I have slithered into the second half of Wilde's/Wotton's formulation, needing my senses cured by my soul.[28]

But please, Lord, not just yet.

---

28   Wait for it. The next line veers into St. Augustine. All of which is to say that you can take the boy out of the Catholic Church, but I think you know the rest.

Mine has become the world of small things.[29] A kind word, a flirty look, a plump khaki-clad ass.
  A globule of cholesterol.

---

29   When I was a teenager, the pastor of the Southern Baptist Church we went to (my father wanting religion but not Catholicism, contra my Catholic-raised mother—long story, another time) gave me a copy of a short book by J. B. Phillips, *Your God Is Too* Small, originally published in 1953 and, I believe, still available today through a press called Touchstone. Subtitled "A Guide for Believers and Skeptics Alike," the book, written by an Anglican canon, encourages its readers to reconsider how they conceive of God, shucking off old labels and conceptions, and redefining the divinity as capable of meeting the needs, challenges, dilemmas, and problems of a complex modern world. Or some such. What has stuck with me is the title. I frequently replace "God" in the title with other conceptual categories. Like "dreams." I also wonder if our God is *too big*—so big that we overlook the small. Perhaps I don't feel like I have much of a choice in thinking this right now.

Small things, but also a phase shift. Time and space. We can never think them separately, or we only ever do so at our peril.

On one hand, everything is slower. On the other hand, my death races toward me much faster than before. I try to compensate by sitting quietly. I take my cup of coffee from Victor and find a cushioned chair. He seemed busy today, rushing from one end of the counter to another, calling out orders for pickup.

I want to be still.

If, reduced to small things, I make myself *also* small, perhaps time will move right past me, not noticing, and everything will just go on and on.

While we were in Colorado, we visited with my dear friend Jane, whom I hadn't seen in years and years. We sat in her living room less than twenty-four hours before my incident.

I called her a few weeks later and told her what had happened. "Get the fuck out of here. What the fuck?"

"Yes, I know."

". . ."

"I know."

"We are all subject to flukes."

"I know."

We got off the phone.

We are all subject to flukes.

But are we? I think she's right, but I have a hard time convincing myself. This can't entirely be a fluke, even if the doctors say so.

There are no guarantees. Okay. But I can't help but wonder if I deserved this somehow.

And then, I think, *what Puritanism, what calculus of divine justice, what foreordained judgment—what self loathing wants me to blame myself?*[30]

---

30   You might have noticed this—". . ."—a couple of times. I unapologetically have stolen ". . ." from the novels of Ronald Firbank. ". . ." is remarkably handy.

Do you think any of this is what I wanted, that any of this is what any one of us would have wanted?

My mother asked a similar question as we waited years and years ago while my sister was in surgery having a cancerous tumor removed. "She didn't want this. She didn't want any of this." Of course not. And neither do I.

And yet, maybe we did, deep down? Maybe we felt we deserved this?

And yet I still need to think of it all as a *gift*. A thing I didn't want but that nonetheless arrived, asking me to figure out what to do with it, what shelf to display it on, what place of honor to give it so that I might show it off when friends come visit.

This is the turn I struggle with.

The night before my incident, or, more precisely, the night *of* the incident, I had a dream. I'm surprised later that I remember the dream, given everything that happened. I would've thought that the trauma of the experience might have so backgrounded my dreamscape that I wouldn't have remembered it.

But I did. I do.

I dreamed that I was in a room and an alligator approached, threatening. I wrestled the alligator to the ground and then jumped on its back and flew it around the room, as though it had transformed into a dragon, tamed at my hands.

I don't know what else to say about this dream.

Perhaps it was both warning and advice. The wild thing, the threat, approaches. *Ride it out, motherfucker. Ride it out.*

Lauren Berlant famously writes about the
fast pace, the crunching out of private time,
the reduction of time and space into a flat
thinness, scooping out the depth of everything.
Everything is so sped up as we hurtle toward the
apocalypse; we rarely have time to think about
what's going on.

In *Cruel Optimism*, Berlant identifies such
contemporary affect as a kind of "slow death," the
steady accumulation of somatic and psychic nicks
and cuts that over a lifetime make life less livable,
or ultimately lethal. Surely some people in parts
of the world live near toxic dumps that are killing
them more quickly than not. But Berlant wants
to attune us to the ways in which corporate
capitalism is producing a culture that might not
be killing us quickly but that is surely killing us
over time.[31]

I recognize how I've been in such a hurry,
there's so much to do, and a quick burger seems
so tempting. But that fast food is slow death. I
have a history of putting in my mouth my own
slow death. I can admit that, looking back on my
life.

And then I think, no, no: I'm not experiencing
slow death. Or maybe I am, but now also

---

31   Lauren Berlant's *Cruel Optimism* was published by Duke
University Press in 2011. Google calls the book "essay."

something else, something different, a different temporality playing fugally alongside my otherwise slow death. It's slow toxicity with the threat of *sudden* death or serious incapacitation, as though a steady diet of harm reaches a critical mass that clogs, chokes, stops the flow within you, the flow that *is* you.

That blocks your ability even to see what's killing you.

If I were to go completely blind, I would miss
the male gaze. My own but also the one at times
directed at me. Seeing it. Feeling it.

I have only recently, within the last few years,
at my advanced age (I'm in my fifties), begun
to notice how I'm noticed in ways that aren't
always hostile, but somehow appreciative, even
momentarily desirous. I have allowed myself to
notice that I, too, am cruised at times. For so long,
I was blinded to such a vision of myself–someone
who could be cruised–made blind by a culture,
an upbringing, a politics, a religion that taught
me I was not worthy: not just not worthy to have
what I desired but, more damagingly, not worthy
to be desired by anyone else.

Not worthy. Not by another man. Not by a boy
I loved. Not in ways that might have saved my
life.

I see now how this damage took part of my
life. It stole time from me. It robbed me of my
youth, much of my young adulthood.

But it also planted within me the invitation
to self-soothe with rich food, to medicate myself
with friendlier spirits, the intoxicants that poison
my blood, that coat the insides of my vessels with
bits of fear and pain. Bits that loosen at times,
unleashing histories of damage I'd almost talked
myself into forgetting.

So it may now be stealing part of my old age.

Not all is toxicity, I remind myself.

I learned to play the piano as a boy, early teens, taking to the instrument readily. I had some talent. I was soothed by my playing, exploring serious music, feeling myself something of an outsider with my love of the classics, but holding to their beauty, relishing even at times the outsider sensation.

I'm different, yes. Possibly even better, *I'd tell myself.*

My feelings matured, thankfully, and, after decades gone by, I still love music and play duets and trios with friends. Susan on the flute, Sue on the upright bass. Wonderful moments, making music, making friendship.

I was scared to play the piano after my incident. Would I be able to see the music? I can still read books, focusing on one line at a time, but reading music requires that you be able to see not just what's directly in front of you, the notes you are playing in that moment, but the notes coming up ahead, a peripheral part of your vision that will turn into future sound.

I wait a couple of months and then go over to Susan's with a bottle of wine. We sit down to play, her flute at the ready, a couple of glasses of wine already in.

I can see just enough to stumble through some new, simple music. There are mistakes, surely. Some misjudgment because I can't quite make out all the upcoming notes. But I can make out enough of them, intuit most of the ones I'll need.

This hasn't been taken from me just yet.

I go home, thinking I might cry, but don't.

I am surprised I am not more angry. And then I am, viciously so.

I shock myself. I sit in rooms, I sit with friends, I barely contain myself, I want to lash out, I want to fucking lash out at everyone around me.

I don't lash out. At least I don't *think* I do. I seethe instead. I seethe inside. This can't be good for my blood pressure. But that may be why I have pills.

I finally take a Xanax at night, a Xanax that the doctor didn't want to give me. Fuck the doctor. Fuck this pill.

Fuck all of you, I think as I go to sleep, wondering if I will wake up.

And then, no.

No, I want you to make demands of me. You, sitting across from me, my friend out with me today, having a "work date," writing down your own thoughts, struggling with your own futurity, your interior sense of where you should be going, what you should be doing.

It's what I like most about you at times. Your earnestness about yourself is beautiful. And then, surprise, you make room for me, make time for me, invite me into your struggle.

I am grateful.

And then I want you to make demands of me. Yes, yes, *you–you* care for me. *You* make time, *you* invite me in. I'm not too crippled yet. The damage has only gone so far.

Make me useful to you yet. Make demands of me.[32]

---

32   I'm stealing these lines from a conversation with a friend I love too much. I'm never not moved when I remember this conversation, the too much love, the too muchness that I need sometimes just to remember that I'm still here.

The beauty of men's bodies. I think of this so often now. I think of my own body, not beautiful, too big, too chunky at points, too pear like. And then I think, *no, I too am beautiful.* I stand in front of the mirror in my bathroom, clad only in my white briefs, looking at myself from different angles. *I am beautiful. Someone will love this body. Someone does.*

I should love this body.

Many of us only have this diminished sense of self, of our bodies, to work with. Many women, surely. Many people of color. But also many queers, even many queer men, queer men of color. Mainstream gay culture doesn't help us much here. Everyone's too pretty, too built, too perfect. Too often white.

I am not perfect. Less so now than ever before. I already have to contend with psychic damage from homophobia. Now I have to contend with the insults of age and the assault of a tiny bit of cholesterol that had ambitions of going out with a bang.

And on some days, I *do.* I *do* contend.

I'm thinking of my dear friend Michelle, someone late in life diagnosed with multiple sclerosis, right when her life was truly coming together, personally, professionally. So many stories I could tell about dear, dear Michelle. But one is playing in my mind right now, over and over.

I'm sitting with Michelle as she's talking to a group of doctors in a medical school, She's been invited to give a talk and answer questions about what it's like to live with MS. She talks about the pills, about mood–altering meds, about antidepressants that help her feel better but also take away much of her sex drive.

"What the doctors don't realize is that, as a lesbian, if you take away my sex drive, I don't really want to live. You're actually not helping me."

Maybe not just lesbians feel this way, but surely, surely, for us queers, can anything be more spot on? I am not only, and Michelle herself is not only, a sex drive. But how dare you try to take it away from us? How dare my own body try to take it away from me? How dare my own body slow me down. And these pills, how dare they.

And then the 2 a.m. erection again. I reach down and hold myself.

I hold myself.

This is the sweetest thing Mack does.

In the morning, getting up right after I do,
as though he's waiting for me to make the first
move, to make sure I'm OK, asking how I slept–
right after we get out of bed and piss, he then
makes his side of the bed and then my side of the
bed, the bed that will wait, ready, made, for us to
return to later that night.

Before, before the incident, before the aftermath, one of my closest friends and I started getting together to make collages. We saved old magazines and books, stuff we were going to recycle or throw out, and decided that we could DIY them into homemade art. A bottle of wine eased the creative process.

Many of these "pieces," which we hang on the walls or set on bookshelves in our homes, are like the adult version of drawings pinned up on the refrigerators of our childhoods. They are pretty negligible as "art." Mashed-up doodles. Colorful miscellany. Inelegantly juxtaposed bric-a-brac. But we love them anyway. They speak of friendship, time shared.

A couple of collages start to become meaningful. I call one my "Hockney Box," composed of images from David Hockney's paintings mixed up with pornographic images from the mid-century physique pictorials that inspired the artist.

The naked men cluster around a Hockney L.A. swimming pool.

I set the box on my living room coffee table, and curious guests' eyes bulge if they happen to open it up.

I don't want to overstate the aesthetic value of this work. I don't actually want to assert any such value at all. But I like the bulging eyes. And I like the seeing and re-seeing that collaging has given us.

And the wine. And the friendship of making together.

I'm turning more and more to such sentiments, to sentimentality itself. Even before the incident. And now, even more so.

My edges bleed.

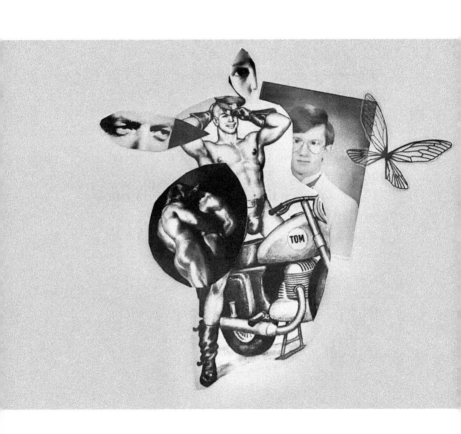

Another collage, lots of pinks and golds, some reds. Naked figures, cut out of magazines. Large eyes, more eyes, drag queen eyes, popping out with color. And then some shiny paper in the background, reflecting paper, so that when you look closely at the assembled images you might also see yourself staring back at you.

The eyes have it. They always do. Not only, but always.

And these collages, reused materials, interrupting the cycle of accumulation and disposal, they also delight. I delight, in their thingness.

I know already that I'm asking too much of them. I'm asking for too much.

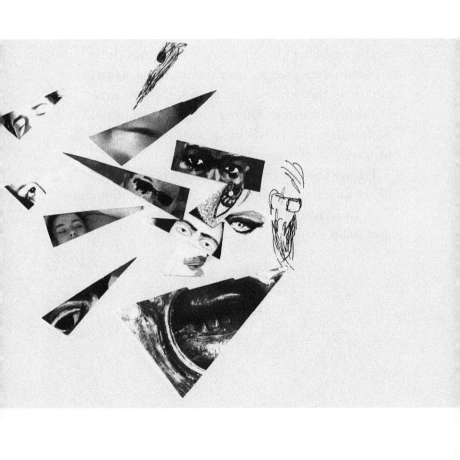

My earliest collages I made in college, in graduate school. I cut out some multicolored triangles, speckled with bright stripes, then some turquoise triangles, pointed and sharp. I spread them out randomly over a piece of white poster paper and put a picture of a cute young man, bespectacled, in the middle. I glued them all down and then spewed white glue all over the triangles, in large circles, as though I'd cum all over the collage.

I called it "Closer Than a Brother" from an old Bible verse: "There is a friend that is closer than a brother."[33]

I don't know where that collage wound up, likely a victim of time, travel, movement, moving.

But I remember so much of it. I close my eyes and see it.

---

33   Again, you can find this on your own. Do you mind if I preserve—the time? the attention? the desire?—of what I look at? It's enough to circulate, yet again, these lines from a devastating book.

So much of our life seems to be about navigating, perhaps even mitigating the rush of the visual, a very sighted person's "problem." How do we make sense of the input, but perhaps more pointedly, how do we learn to pay attention to what *needs* our attention, while not turning a completely blind eye to what's left, what might be approaching out of the corner, what might be sneaking up on us?

I want a genealogy of this attunement of the eyes, this visual training.[34]

But for now, I also want to make collages that are about a spectacle of sight, a mishmash, not just an assemblage, but a raucous accumulation, a conglomeration of things.

My Hockney box, for instance, jam–packed with images from the artist's paintings of nude men mixed in with actual porn. I cut out the naked bodies and arrange them, cocks at attention, around a shiny bit of blue. A Hockney

---

34   Sarah Ahmed, in *Queer Phenomenology*, published by Duke University Press in 2006, talks about the power of orientation and disorientation to direct and redirect attention. Some of us are situated differently; that is, we are oriented in the world so that our vision, our attention, falls on things outside the norm. This *queer* orientation offers critical insight into the order of things, their arrangement, and the normative paths laid out to navigate them. Critical, that is, if you can survive your own dis–orientation.

pool party, the boys come home to play. It's an extravaganza of pornographic images.

A conglomeration. So much to look at. So much still to see.

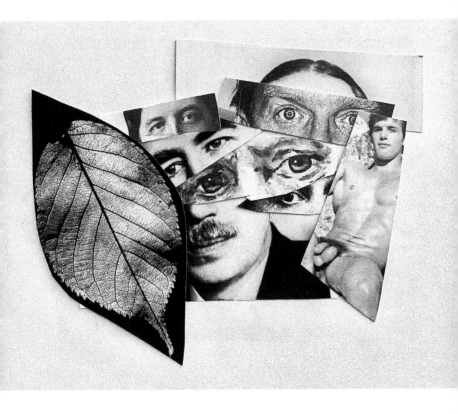

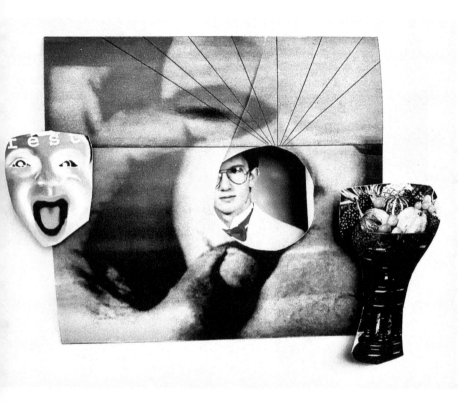

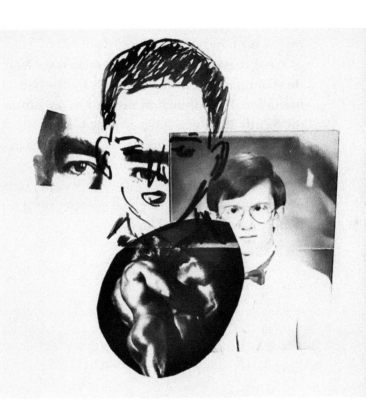

You must change your life. Rilke.

You, reader, you must know it.[35] The poet looking at a statue, the torso of Apollo. Isn't this the highest aesthetic education–the call made by the work of art for us to be other than what we are, more than the given, however less than the divine for which we might strive?

What makes up the moments when we feel this command from without, this more-than-an invitation, this injunction not just to do, but to do differently than you have already?

What are those moments? What changes in a moment?

I see myself reflected in the shiny paper of my own collages. No one else will see this, but I know that I must change my life.

Again.

---

35   And if you don't, here it is, "Archaic Torso of Apollo," translated by Stephen Mitchell, on poets.org: https://poets.org/poem/archaic-torso-apollo.

I'm constantly checking in with myself. This is not new. I've done this as long as I can remember. "How are you doing?" I ask myself. Usually early in the morning, perhaps when I'm sitting on the toilet, or in the midst of making coffee.

(I think of Victor sometimes, and his khaki-clad bottom, when I'm making coffee at home. Not every time, but sometimes. Is he too making coffee while I am?)

The answer is, usually, "I'm fine. I'm okay." Sometimes it's "I'm angry." I've often been angry in the past. I'm angry sometimes now.

Indeed, increasingly, with time, more often than not now, it's "I'm angry." But I quickly tell myself, "No, you aren't angry. You aren't. You're okay. Really."

"I'm fine." Until I'm not.

I start a lot of books right now.

I've always read several books at one time, sometimes as many as twelve or thirteen books, my nightstand a repository for reading–in–progress. Periodically I commit to finishing several at once, and spend consecutive evenings going through them one by one, finishing book after book. Then the pile of reading–in–progress starts to accumulate again.

Binge and purge.

Right now, though, I'm just starting books. I haven't finished a book in weeks. I just keep starting them, one after another. I want to go to the bookstore or library every day to find a new book to start. I look forward to the starting, over and over again.

I don't want to complete any of them. Not right now.

The flows, the paths, the wrong turn, the devastation.

I write out this sequence and realize that it implies–it even *asserts*–the activity of agency at some point. We're flowing along and then make a choice, perhaps not entirely consciously, but just enough to open up the question of culpability when we arrive at the scene of devastation.

I have arrived. I have questions.

One of my dearest friends, someone who has devoted her life to the study of the classical world, characterizes my incident as an act of divine intervention. But for her, the intervention is a *smiting* and, given her deep affinity for the ancient pagans, a smiting without meaning. Not every act of the gods needs to be understandable, or have a human reason.

"It's like the hand of god came down and smote you."

For her, the question is answered. The smiting is sufficient unto itself.

I look for other answers. It's inevitable. Who wouldn't, except my classically oriented friend, and perhaps other pagans resigned (or so they say) to the fateful vicissitudes of unpredictable life?

I am obsessed for a while with searching for
articles, images, videos, anything that describes
how animals, dogs and cats mostly, see.

What does the world look like to them?

I gaze on images of muddied backgrounds,
blindspots, grayed–out areas, bits and pieces that,
with a human eye, would resolve into some kind
of clarity.

I wonder if I am becoming more animal.

This morning walking to work, misty with a bit
of a chill in the air, I feel my briefs cupping my
ass, the swish of khaki fabric between my legs
as I strut briskly to work. My ass pumps out
the strides, one after another, and I feel myself
animal, stalking the sidewalk.

I am powerful.

I could keep going like this, animal, pumping,
my behind working out this walk to work.

Some days I avoid writing these thoughts. I work on other things, administrative memos, an academic article. Something that we call "productive."[36]

But not these thoughts, not these words.

I want, instead, to dwell in the present of my own ongoingness, the work I am doing, the already entered and seemingly ceaseless conversations.

On those days, I turn away from the diary. I don't want to think these other thoughts, these recognitions of imminent cessation. I write otherwise, writing my way out of them, for now.

---

36   Eric Michaels's *Unbecoming* is instructive about avoidance and the pressure of productivity, even as the author recounts dying of AIDS. What kind of world do we live in? What kind of world pressures the dying to feel productive?

The best days, I swear, are the ones in which, often at a moment in the afternoon when I reach a lull in my work or whatever I'm doing, I just sit back and think, *I'm so lucky, I'm so grateful, this is it, this is all there needs to be.* I quickly think, *no, I'm lying, there's more, so much more I want.*

But I force myself to take the moment to feel the gratitude. I'm not always sure where it comes from. I know it won't last.

I still think those are the best days.

Four months in, I go to the optometrist. I need new glasses. Normally, before the incident, if the incident had never happened, this would be the time for me to think about new frames, something stylish. This time, though, new *lenses*.

I sit in the chair, the doctor comes in, glad to see me. I tell her what's been going on. She is, of course, concerned. She dilates my eyes, wants to take a look. She looks, she wants to see it for herself. She's curious. She's even fascinated.

She sees it, the globule, bright yellow.

"Oh no, not your good eye," she says.

I feel myself so permeable right now. I am not solid. I wonder at times if you could see through me.

No, I don't wonder that. I exaggerate. Even my sense of my own permeability isn't stable, isn't solid.

I have written elsewhere against the idea of legacy. I do not have children. My books will not be read by many, increasingly no one. I will not be remembered. I'm OK with this. I'd rather accept this than fight against it.

Time does not just permeate us. It shreds us.

No. Sometimes I just want to say *no*.
Or I wake up and ask myself how I feel.
"I'm angry."
I don't know why I say this.
No.
Just *no*.

This is what my plaque looks like. This is my incident.

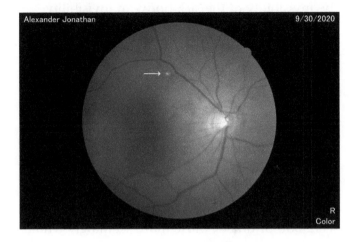

Again, Maia Dolphin-Krute, this time writing in *Ghostbodies: Towards a New Theory of Invalidism*, about the invisibility of the sick body, an invisibility which starts to seem to her like a ghosting, something not quite seen by others, or caught only out of the corner of one's eyes.[37]

Something ghosted by others. Others who don't want to see the damaged, the incapacitated, the invalid, the in-valid.

I get it. My damage becomes ghostly, after the shock and the kind words. *Oh my god. That's awful.* And then back to normal. I see it, my damage, all the time, or I see the absence of what is no longer seen. But for others, those more seemingly whole than I am now, this damage is the thing not just barely seen, but the thing not *wanted* to be seen.

It's ghosted. I'm ghosted.

But Maia reminds me: "Loss is not an inherently negative sensation."

Indeed. I sense the ghosted part of me, the damage that has made an absence. And then I feel the ghosting of others, their all too understandable unwillingness to live in a world of constant damage.

---

37   *Ghostbodies: Towards a New Theory of Invalidism* was published by the University of Chicago Press in 2017. The direct quotation appears on page 57.

Their unwillingness isn't a "negative sensation."
It's palpable, a presence.

I am afraid to fly. I used to fly monthly, going
to different conferences, giving talks, mostly for
work. Always for work. Rarely just for pleasure.
But I'd learned over time to build in pleasurable
activities during my work trips. Sometimes
I'd stay an extra day or two. At times, I admit,
traveling so much became a drag. Especially with
age, it can be hard on the body.

But I did it. I like feeling busy, in motion.
Movement. Space as time. Time measured in
distances traveled, experiences gained, things
seen.

Things *seen.*

Now I worry, despite people telling me not
to, that the differential air pressure while flying
might lodge something else loose. Something
*un*seen. Things unseen that will still transform my
life into another incident, another aftermath.

If I survive them.

I have taken to wearing a scarf, usually one purchased at a museum shop.

Admittedly, the effect is a bit femme, but I like it, perhaps *because* it is femme. I bought my first scarf with my "opera friend," a woman I travel to see operas with. I know, I know, it's so pretentious. Except we're not pretending: We really do love opera, a taste I've developed relatively late in life.

On one such trip, my first after the incident, we flew up to San Francisco to see a production of Benjamin Britten's *Billy Budd*. I'd seen the opera before, but so many years ago that a repeat experience seemed warranted, especially given my current interest in opera. And besides, it's an all-male opera about a guy who wants to destroy the young men he's in love with but can't bring himself to admit that he's in love with. It's an astonishing piece, with a libretto by E. M. Forster of all people.

This was a "big trip" for me–only an hour away, but one that still felt like taking a chance, going out of town, spending the night somewhere else, risking waking up to a terrifying loss of vision. But I felt it was something that had to be done.

While in the Bay Area, we also checked out a museum that had an exhibit of the tattoo work of Ed Hardy. Lots and lots of tattooed flesh, including of intimate parts. I thrilled especially to a pair of tattooed male buttocks, which were already perfectly shaped and now adorned with colorful swirls and stripes. Exquisite.

But the major find of the exhibit was a scarf with one of Hardy's tattoo designs on it, a black panther on red and blue background. Also exquisite. I had to have it. My friend taught me how to make a Parisian knot, but made me promise we wouldn't wear our scarves (she bought an identical one) to the same function. Apparently that's a no-no.

I only realized later that this scarf, and the others I've bought and worn, are wrapped around my neck, around one of the arteries from which a little piece of plaque likely broke off and lodged in my eye. I'm protecting my neck–purely psychologically, because it's never cold enough (to me) in Southern California to warrant a scarf.

But I wear them anyway.

The pile of books by the side of my bed continues to accumulate, more now than ever before. So many books. I continue to start them, and then set them aside for another and another.

I still don't want any of them to end.

I put a picture of the stack of books on Facebook and someone commented, insightfully, that I have built a barricade on my side of the bed. A wall, a shelter made of books.

Books I won't complete. But books that signal potential, worlds opening.

The usual.

Everyone talks about a wake-up call, but can you know what that is until you hear it yourself?

Everything I write here is almost cliché, I think, except when it becomes granular, when you're living it yourself. None of it is cliché to me. The sacred smallness of things.

But there it is. The cliché.

And then I pick up a book, read memoirs of those whose marriages fall apart because of sudden illness, quick catastrophe, the damage that strikes without warning. Unions dissolve. Partners split. They have no more time for what they thought they wanted.

Christine Hyung-Oak Lee writes about her marriage in *Tell Me Everything You Don't Remember: The Stroke That Changed My Life.*[38] She does right by her husband, who tried to stay with her through the difficult times, the post-stroke life that robbed Christine of so much memory, so much past. But how could he, the husband, make a future without enough of a past, a past she couldn't always remember?

He couldn't. But *she* still had to. With whatever time she has left.

---

38   *Tell Me Everything You Don't Remember: The Stroke That Changed My Life*, a heartbreaking book I can barely stand to read at times, was published by Ecco Press in 2017. (I'm beginning to think that 2017 was a really good year for books about damage.)

What kind of future comes from having no more time for what you thought you wanted?

Sometimes I want to make up stories about different bodily oddities, like the diagonal wrinkle across my forehead. It is actually diagonal. I have no idea how it got there. It cuts across the other more horizontal wrinkles that have steadily been appearing over the last decade.

Where does it come from?

It was perhaps the first wrinkle I really noticed. So strange. My very own Harry Potter lightning bolt, but I don't know what history it tells, what time past it represents, pushing its way out of my body into a crevice.

Time, shredding me, refusing to disclose its secrets.

There may be no secret.

But I refuse to believe that. There are always stories. There are always stories that we tell, and not just to make sense of what's happened. That's the *least* level of storytelling, the least way in which stories emerge, viral, permeating us like time.

Stories *are* time.

Stories are the technology that we use to *change* time. It is not sufficient to just explain. We spew out stories, like a contagion, wanting to infect what *comes next.*

Here's another story.

My friend Elizabeth, my great friend from college with whom I steadily lost contact after we graduated, who stayed behind in Baton Rouge after I'd left for Colorado, then Ohio, then California, a husband, a queer life. My friend Elizabeth, whom I depended on, with whom I commiserated, with whom I struggled to understand the role that religion would and ultimately would not play in my life, my friend with whom I made hard choices about growing up.

So much to say here. But I'll say this. We rarely talked after college. In the last twenty years, I saw her twice, once in California, once in Louisiana, both on occasions in which one of us was just passing through. Sometimes a text, or Facebook message. But no sustained conversation. And that was OK, I think, on both ends. We had done what we needed to do, and helped launch each other into the rest of our lives.

Then, during the weekend of my incident, she started calling. I missed a few calls from her, out of the blue. We were busy that weekend, checking out properties, so I didn't call back. I sent a text. "What's up?" I didn't hear back, and then the incident happened.

At one point, she left a message.

"Pinecone."

That was it. One word. An inside joke I won't tell you about. But I will tell you that I smiled.

And then, a month later, she's dead. Kidney and liver failure. Just two years older than I am.

I think she knew she was dying and wanted to connect. I could be angry that my incident focused my attention so much on myself that I missed that chance. But I'm warmed by the thought that, toward the end, she thought of me. I wish I could've told her that I was thinking of her too. I was.

I am.

I think that, queer, I experience time differently. Not all queers will feel their way through time the way I do, but my queerness, my choice not to reproduce, my insistence on cultivating intergenerational relationships, my primary relationship with its relative lack of markers of "maturity"–all are stakes on time but with a difference. Nonnormative time. Non-heteronormative time.

So I don't know, perhaps, how to die. I don't know, that is, how to die like others will die, are dying, have died. I don't know what my death will look like.

And surely, who does? But my friend, an older friend, straight, one thinking about her own death, must know that her death will likely be surrounded by her kids, her grandkids, her blood relatives easing her passing.

Who will be with us when we die? Who will ease my passing, Mack's passing?

Who will help us spend that time until there's no more time?

And then the odd moment, always the odd moment, that allows such thoughts to pass from my mind into the beauty of the present.

I'm riding down in the elevator and a construction worker, young, Latino, hops on the elevator with me. (The construction work on the outside of this building seems interminable.)

I'm texting a friend, but I feel the worker looking at me, checking me out. *Am I being cruised?* I think.

I look up from my phone and he smiles.

"I have lunch at 11."

Really? I think, but can't help but be pleased.

"I hope you enjoy your lunch," I say as I step off the elevator, giving him my own smile that I hope shows him only my gratitude.

We have decided to become vegan. I think this is the kind of thing that happens when you've had an incident. You are given an opening, a window, a time to make big changes.

This is a big change.

My cholesterol was already pretty much under control (except for the obvious bit that wasn't), so deciding just to go ahead and eliminate it from my diet seems a radical choice.

I don't mind being radical.

But even so, sometimes you need a push to do the radical thing. And then again, is it really *that* radical, what we're doing? Is this a surrogate radicality? Is this a thing I can do and *feel* radical, when in fact there are more drastic, more devastatingly radical things I could be doing?

I will admit that I like the comforts of being ideological. I could easily become an ideological vegan. Anthony Bourdain once called vegans the Hezbollah–like sect of the vegetarians.[39] I was sitting on the toilet when I first read that and started laughing so uproariously that Mack came running to see if something was wrong.

Nothing wrong. Just identification.

---

39   Bourdain says this in *Kitchen Confidential: Adventures in the Culinary Underbelly*. His suicide is still with me. We spent the summer after his death watching his television shows. We imagined we could see his unraveling. But whom are we kidding? Who can ever see an unraveling, except the person being shredded?

I train to Fullerton for the day to sit in a coffee shop and write. I break for lunch and allow myself to pull some attitude at a restaurant that says it has vegan options but *really, what the fuck,* doesn't. Seriously.

So yes, I'm going to allow myself to pull some attitude. I can't help but feel that I deserve it.

We are ready to save the planet when we have some skin in the game. Or at least that's what we tell ourselves: *We're going vegan because it's environmentally friendly.*

That's what we're doing: saving the planet, one meal at a time.

Sometimes we are just so full of shit.

Even in writing this, I realize I am confronting how judgmental I can be. Not complaining, mind you. Confronting, which is also, in my world, a form of appreciating.

I can appreciate a good judgment.

Once, with Mack, in Amsterdam, at the Rijk's Museum, walking past some famous Van Gogh, Mack saw an old woman taking a flash photograph of one of the priceless paintings. Without hesitation, he walked up to her and started chastising her. A friend of ours looked away with embarrassment. I just started grinning, delighted, even a tiny bit aroused.

Knowing better, ah the comforts of *knowing better* and the world consequently becoming full of teachable moments. I sound like an asshole. And sometimes both Mack and I can be assholes. *But it's for your own good*, we say.

Justification, rationalization, identification. I could easily become an ideological vegan. I want to feel certain, convinced, a believer.

I want to feel sure.

And then I remember: *Probabilities are not guarantees.*

What do I, really, know? And how far can the smug superiority of turning vegan really take me?

Everything is still slower. Almost five months in, and I walk around my campus, moving from one meeting to another, and I'm overwhelmed by the feeling that it will take me forever to get from one building to another. A quarter mile of eternity.

I'm still not (mostly) complaining. When I talk about this sometimes to others, they think I'm bitching about it, disgruntled that I've been *slowed down*. But I'm mostly good with it, the slowing down, even just the sensation that, somehow, to use a disgraced word, I've been *retarded*.

I can't quite let go of that word. It reminds me of the music term: *ritardando*. Slowing down. My phenomenological experience of the world, even now, well over four months in, is *ritardando*.[40]

---

40 Phenomenology is what happens after the fall, when we are kicked out of the garden, when we can no longer assume the divine penetration and justness of every thing around us. It is when we have to start paying attention. It is when the world has grown strange.

José Esteban Muñoz says, "To access queer
visuality, we may need to squint, to strain our
vision and force it to see otherwise, beyond the
limited vista of the here and now."[41]

Now I squint, quite literally.

I squint, therefore I'm queer.

And I thought I was queer *before*.

---

41   This quotation appears on page 22 of *Cruising Utopia:*
The Then and There of Queer Futurity, published by New York
University Press in 2009. This book is definitely "self-help," no
matter what Google says.

I pause with Muñoz to think about what's queer about my story.

I can't answer that question without approaching a different but related question: *What's my relationship to my body?*

This is the question around which my queerness emerges, does its work, announces itself. This body marked me from the beginning, a little bit sissy, just a tad femme. Other. Not normal.

Not. Just not.

This is the knot of knowledge untied by the queer, because it's never just my body being *not*. It's always my body in relation to other bodies. So queer becomes less the thing *I am* and more the thing *I am called to be and can't quite manage. The thing I fail at being. The excess of that failure.* And then that failure becomes the story I start to tell about myself, the one I have spent the remainder of my life trying to tell differently, but always in relation to the stories that others are telling, the story initially given to me about me and my body, so not normal.

Oh, all the questions others demanded I ask of myself: *Am I too much like a girl? Am I too fey? Do I lisp too much?* But also, *am I not gay enough? Am I too fat? Are my eyes too crossed? Am I too bald?*

I remember meeting some gay colleagues at a work function, some professors at our law school

I'd never met before. We exchanged pleasantries, but I could feel their assessing eyes looking me up and down. We talked about the catering, a local restaurant, a new local favorite. I expressed some hesitation, some ambivalence. *Meh*, I said.

"Are you even really gay?" One of the lawyers nearly shrieked this accusation. How could I not like this restaurant if I'm *actually* gay?

Again, my body betrays me. What I taste, how I taste, my *tastes* don't fit in. But again, always in relation, always in the presence of others who are looking, assessing, until that seeing becomes part of the story I tell myself, part of how I see myself. Part of how I *taste*.

I'm always trying to interrupt that seeing, block it, blind myself to it a little bit so that I can see for myself, if such a thing is even, so belatedly, possible.

Are you even really gay?

I guess what's queer about my story is how I've never not been aware of this play of looking over bodies, no matter who's looking, straight or gay, faggot or not.

And maybe now I'm starting to care about who's looking *just a little bit less.*

I walk down the hall from my office to the bathroom to take a piss. After locking the door, I drop my pants and briefs, position myself in front of the urinal, arch my back to stretch, and start to urinate. I've had a lot of water this morning, and I delight in the strong stream as it hits the porcelain. I arch my back further, feeling my animal self enjoy a good piss.

I wonder how much longer I'll be able to enjoy this. Could this be my last good piss? Do I walk out of this bathroom into an incident later today that will take from me this simple pleasure?

As with so much of my life before, I'm re-orienting: doing something different, challenging myself with new ways of being in the world.

Going vegan. Making collages. Re-learning to read, read music. Trying to learn how to fly and not succumb to panic. Enjoying a good piss more than ever before.

I am never far from the call to orient, to re-orient, to begin again.[42]

You must change your life.[43]

---

42   See earlier note on Ahmed.

43   See earlier note on Rilke. It's at this point that I'm starting to accrue an orientation. I know that's a mixed metaphor, but "accrue" seems like just the right word (even though my auto-correct wants to change it to "accuse.")

Mack and I go to our new favorite vegan restaurant.

Each new vegan restaurant is our favorite one. There are so many in Southern California, so hip here, that we'll have favorites, I feel, for some time to come.

We enjoy the meal, a bottle of vegan wine, in this cafe in a hipster shopping complex called, pretentiously, The Lab. Avo tacos, mushroom chorizo, pickled everything. All served by young people in black in a space cramped enough to be on the Left Bank. We're loving it.

Mack sits against the wall, hung with large posters of young people cavorting on the beach. So Southern California. Even though we hardly ever go to the beach (as most of our friends don't either), we are constantly being reminded that we live right next to the ocean.

My eye—one of them, both of them trading off—keeps looking up to the poster over Mack's head: two boys, three girls jumping up in the air, hands raised to the sky, their feet just leaving the hot sand. All thin, all tanned, all healthy. One boy in particular catches my eye, his shirt just rising above his belly button as he reaches up, up, revealing not only his navel but the gray waistband of his underpants.

I keep looking, looking back at that waistband. It leads my eye on, as the pose intended.

This much still works.

I'm overtaken at times by questions of what I do and do not want to do again. For instance, Mack asks me, "Do you want to try to drive again?"

My car, the one I most often drove, sits outside our house. Mack takes it for a spin about once a week, so it won't feel lonely or neglected, I think.

"We could get you a driving instructor that specializes in working with people who have lost some sight . . ."

Mack is so sweet. But I'm just not sure. I don't know. I don't know if I want to drive again. I don't know if I want to learn how to drive again.

I just don't know. And I'm going to allow myself to sit with that for a while.[44]

---

44 We eventually sold that car to someone in our neighborhood. We see it around every now and then. Mother once saw it, the bright yellow car, and texted me. I couldn't stop the tears, until I did.

Other questions come, or return, seeming new, renewed.

What life am I crowding out? What aspects of my being languish or remain underdeveloped–or have actually *died*–because I couldn't or didn't attend to them while I was focusing on building myself professionally, cultivating defensively the kind of life of security and moderate prosperity that would signal that there's nothing damaged here, that there's only the good stuff, success, value, pride in a job well done?[45]

What time do I have left for the already crowded out?

And what will still be, despite my best intentions, crowded out?

---

45   I've actually stolen this from another book I'm writing, because it just works well here.

I am kinder to old people. Gentler.
    I talk to them.
    I didn't realize I was already one of them.[46]

---

46   This is a constant refrain of Hervé Guibert in *The Compassion Protocol*. Some are old, become old, long before they are due. Guibert's book was published in English in 1993 by Quartet Books and seems now, unfortunately, out of print.

The last year of my father's life was a total shitshow.

My mother was trapped in the house with him, serving as his primary caretaker. My heart broke for her. I visited as often as I could, listened to her misery, took my father to doctors for check-ins, and, late one night, pried her off him. He'd pissed the bed, again, and woken her up to clean his mess.

"You've ruined my life. You've ruined my life," she furiously murmured, leaning over his prone body.

I couldn't blame her. I don't blame her. He was, at times, cold, cruel, distant. He left her no money for her own retirement. She lost a solid decade and more of her life having to tend to him and his piss-stained beds.

There's so much more I could say here.

And then I think: *Did this really happen? Did I catch her whispering furiously? Or was that me, me hovering over him, accusing?*

Who doesn't want to have the chance to accuse the one who has ruined your life—even if, to be fair, it is you, it is you, and it is you who will finally pick yourself up after the ruin and begin to live?

Mother, who now lives with us in California, dear mother, sometimes spills things. She's not that old, but sometimes the cup is too heavy. A small mess, easily handled.

I see one of the spills she didn't quite clean completely, just a drop or two of coffee hanging out on the counter, and I start to cry.

Is this what aging is like?

So easy to misjudge the distance, to overreach, under reach, just a glancing past. I have to reorient myself in space to compensate for my blindspot. And I think, seeing my mother's coffee stains, is *this what aging is like?*

Too soon. Always too soon.

All of the thoughts coming at me while I stand in the shower, scribbling in the steam on the glass to try to create a trace in memory.

I watch my words evaporate.

A young man once asked me about being cross–
eyed. He was a teenager. He really didn't know
any better.

"Can you get that corrected?"

"Yes. But I don't want to. It lets me know who
in the world is an asshole, and who isn't."

A year later, a year after the incident, a friend, Karen, who came to see me in the hospital, will ask me if I've acclimated, adjusted, if I've gotten enough back to "normal" that I don't think about my incident in quite the same way as I did in its immediate aftermath.

What she is asking is if I have come once more to take my life for granted.

How can I? How can I when my body has let me know that it could kill me at any moment? How can I take anything I see in the world for granted when I know, every time I open my eyes, that I'm only seeing part of the world I used to be able to see? When every night, in the middle of the night, in the quiet, I still wake up and check to see, *can I see? Am I still here?*

Patrick Anderson, near the end of *Autobiography of an Illness* calls on, or as I'm tempted to say, *summons* the radical theorist Jasbir Puar, someone with her own streak of the destructive, the damage of too many different kinds of aftermath: "This quality of prognosis–enabling storytelling about oneself in an uncertain future–serves a larger purpose than the simplistic promise of singular optimism in the face of debilitating illness or injury: it promotes and demands the eminently social project of *hope*." Or, as Jasbir Puar says, glossing the work of Lisa Duggan, hope is a risk "that must be taken in order to reconfigure the very forms of sociality that produce the dialectic between hope and hopelessness in which we are situated in the first place."[47]

We demand this promise, this hope, that our damages can remake the world. Loss becomes dialectic.

But isn't the mistake in thinking that we have lost anything in the first place? We only lose if we believe that we were promised anything to begin with.

---

47   I love the layering here. Anderson, Duggan, Puar. More accrual. The quotation appears in Puar's article "Prognosis Time: Towards a Geopolitics of Affect, Debility and Capacity," published in volume 19 (2009) of *Women and Performance: A Journal of Feminist Theory* (pages 161–172).

And we are indeed made promises. Life, liberty, the pursuit of happiness.

But no one can make those promises. We are fools to have believed them in the first place.

Some days feel like progress, even if I'm not sure what that means.

Today, I'm sitting across from my favorite hipster, David, a Brooklyn-based writer who's in town for a couple of months, wintering in SoCal. I have a fondness for hipsters, I have to admit. I know, I know, there's much to revile. David had taken me on a walking tour of Brooklyn a couple of years ago, and we expressed great dismay at the gentrification of large parts of this borough, a gentrification that has been pricing many low-income and working-class residents out of their homes for years. More corporate capitalism run amok. David knows that hipsters are part of the problem; their aesthetic, however DIY and remix it might be at times, also signals, like the gays used to, the arrival of the "creative class," and the wealthy always seem to want to be around the "creative class," even if they end up driving the poorer creatives out.

David and I sit across from one another, having just purchased our high-priced coffees at the hipster coffee shop, and while I bemoan the intertwining of hipster aesthetic and gentrification, I have to admit that I enjoyed the fact that it took about twelve minutes for the tattooed barista to make my pour over.

Twelve minutes.

That's nearly the time I spend in meditation every morning. Whatever one might say about hipsters, this attention to detail, to taking one's time, to waiting for a good thing–and the pour overs at this particular coffee shop are totally worth waiting for–that slowness has become deeply attractive to me. It's a ramping down, a pulling back, a moment of respite before I crack open the laptop and get to work.

I need more and more of those moments of respite before I recharge my body for the work ahead. I'm grateful for the hipsters who teach me about such slowness, particularly as I sit across from one who writes for a living, who wonders where his next story opportunity will come from, who lives from word count to word count, pitching his talent to media corporations that otherwise won't hire writers full–time. His own urgency in this economic climate, this increasingly toxic economic reality that makes people so desperately responsible for themselves, is met and momentarily relieved by his willingness to wait with me for that pour over.

Our urgency is put on pause to enjoy something. That feels like progress.

Until it doesn't.

A couple of hours later, I get up from my writing
and walk around the complex, gazing at the little
shops, some selling cheese and spices, others
offering way-too-expensive clothing. I'm not
really looking but daydreaming, taking a break
from clacking away at the laptop. I allow myself
these little strolls because I can only sit at the
computer for about an hour at a time, and then
my body–my damaged eye, the one I still seem to
prefer to read out of–demands that I get up and
move.

So I walk around and think about what else I
have to do today, what I want to make for dinner,
what I want to write in the future, what projects
await, and the walking turns to real dreaming,
picking up on a prolonged meditation that's
always at the back of my mind about where I'm
taking my life, the paths I intend to follow, the
desires I have to make a difference not just in my
life but in the world around me, in the lives of
the people I love, to be there for them, to be there
for those I can't even imagine coming into my life
yet, but who always do.

I've come to appreciate these little daydream
strolls as more than just the body needing a
break. They are the body moving my mind. They
are a little opening onto and into futurity.

The Marxist philosopher Ernst Bloch
understood them as glimmers of utopian

thought and feeling. While our night dreams
confront us with images and situations over
which we have little conscious control, the
refuse of the unconscious mind, our daydreams
are wanderings and wonderings that we can
participate in and actively cultivate.[48]

Bloch rejects the Freudian unconscious, the
no-longer-conscious, the neurotic tendrils of the
past, He rejects them so that we might better
become attuned to traces of the *not-yet-conscious*.
Daydreams are less about repression and what
we fear to make manifest, but instead concern
themselves more with *expression*, a playful
engagement with the longed-for, the barely and
all-too-briefly glimpsed horizon of possibilities.
Bloch sees such horizons nearly everywhere, and
he constructs an aesthetic philosophy that's all

---

48   Bloch put it this way: "The day-dreaming 'I' persists
throughout, consciously, privately, envisaging the
circumstances and images of a desired, better life. . . . It is
concerned with an as far as possible unrestricted journey
forward, so that . . . the images of that which is not yet
can be phantasied into life and into the world." I like that
"phantasied into life and into the world," a possibility that
led Bloch to wonder, "Should one dream . . . only when
one is asleep and not at all when one is awake?" The Bloch
quotations are variously reprinted but can be found on page
87 of *A Philosophy of the Future* (1963; New York: Herder and
Herder, 1970).

about tracing the utopian possibilities latent in most art and culture, including our daydreams. His magnum opus, *The Principle of Hope*, exists as a compendium of such daydreams, pulled from across history and the arts.

For Bloch, utopianism comes from our ability to dream, to *daydream*.

But daydreams take time. We need to *take the time* to entertain them, to welcome them, to cultivate them.

And then, I think, *what time do I have? Will there be time enough, for hope?*

Will there be enough?[49]

---

49   Some of the last two entries (maybe much of it?) is recast from the *LARB* article I mentioned earlier. It just felt right here, and earlier, remixed as it were. Scattered. *Re-seen.*

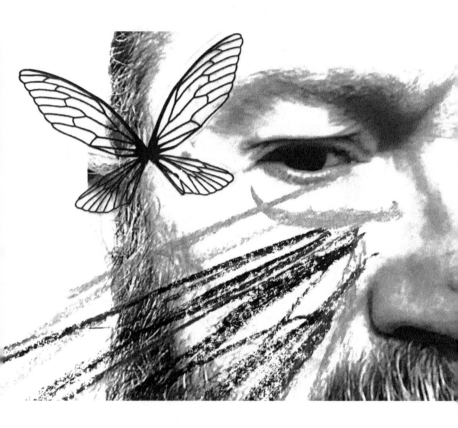

In the morning, before work again, well over a year later, I go to the coffee shop. I've gotten busy, haven't been in a while. It's nice to be back.

More crowded than normal, more activity. I feel myself here, check in with my body. I stretch a little bit, glad of the company, glad of the young folk moving quickly around me. I stand in line, check out the boy in front. Cute. Firm ass. I flex my own buttocks.

Good to be here.

I get to the front of the line, looking up from my phone, the barista all smiles.

But no Victor. Not today.

He doesn't work here anymore.

Acknowledgments

I am grateful to so many people as I think
about this little book's conception, writing,
and publication. Fredric Nachbaur at Fordham
University Press has been a generous and
gracious guide, shepherding the book through
a generative review process and production
period. Teresa Jesionowski and Eric Newman
were extraordinary in guiding me through the
production process. And my two reviewers
offered superb suggestions and recommendations.
Patrick Anderson "outed" himself after submitting
his review so we could continue talking about
queerness and disability, and I'm deeply indebted
to his kind and gentle genius.

Friends and family provided significant
support in the aftermath of my health crisis and
in supporting my ongoing desire to write–about
this and other topics. They are David Lumb,
Karen Yescavage, Sherryl Vint, David Wallace,
Jackie Rhodes, Antoinette LaFarge, Kelly Maloney,
Jack Miles, Katherine Mack, Daniel M. Gross and

Carla Wilson, and Cristina and Tim Garrity. Our
"family," which has been meeting regularly for
dinners for years, basically saved my life: Susan C.
Jarratt, Nasrin Rahimieh, and George Lang joined
me, Mack, and Mother for countless good times
and commiseration during the difficult times.
Susan, comrade, colleague, confidant, has been a
most special friend at this time; she was the first
one with whom I played music after my incident,
me wondering if I could see sufficiently to read a
score.

At UC, Irvine, Jim Lee has been a trusted and
thoughtful interlocutor for some time about the
body and its vicissitudes. Michelle Latiolais has
encouraged my creative nonfiction. Dillon Sefic,
an amazing MFA student with whom I worked
(and a writer you will want to watch out for), was
the first to read the complete manuscript and
offered some of the best advice I received.

Tom Lutz, Eric Newman, and Boris Dralyuk at
the *Los Angeles Review of Books* have been staunch
supporters of my writing, and I am grateful
to them for initially publishing some bits and
pieces that have made their way into this diary.
And I am likewise grateful to Jackie Rhodes who
originally published my thinking about Sarah
Manguso and Maggie Nelson in her special issue
of *Pre/Text*, delightfully called "Dirtysexy" (volume
24, 2018). And finally, obviously, Mack and

Mother–I wouldn't know what to do without you. All my best love–and my worst, I'm afraid. You mean the world to me because you *are* my world.

Works Cited

Ahmed, Sarah. *Queer Phenomenology*. Durham, NC:
   Duke University Press, 2006.

Alexander, Jonathan. *Creep: A Life, a Theory, an
   Apology*. Goleta, CA: punctum books, 2017.

Anderson, Patrick. *Autobiography of a Disease*. New
   York: Routledge, 2017.

Berlant, Lauren. *Cruel Optimism*. Durham, NC: Duke
   University Press, 2011.

Bloch, Ernst. *A Philosophy of the Future*. Translated by
   John Cumming. New York: Herder and Herder,
   1970.

Butler, Judith. *Giving an Account of Oneself*. New York:
   Fordham University Press, 2005.

Dolphin–Krute, Maia. *Ghostbodies: Towards a New
   Theory of Invalidism*. Chicago: University of
   Chicago Press, 2017.

Dolphin–Krute, Maia. *Visceral: Essays on Illness Not as
   Metaphor*. Goleta, CA: punctum books, 2017.

Durbin, Andrew. "Hervé Guibert: Living without a
   Vaccine." *New York Review*, June 12, 2020.

Frank, Arthur W. *The Wounded Storyteller: Body, Illness, and Ethics*. 1995. Chicago: University of Chicago Press, 2013.

Guibert, Hervé. *The Compassion Protocol*. Translated by James Kirkup. New York: George Braziller, 1994.

Guibert, Hervé. *Cytomegalovirus: A Hospitalization Diary*. Translated by Clara Orban. New York: Fordham University Press, 2015.

Guibert, Hervé. *To the Friend Who Did Not Save My Life*. Translated by Linda Coverdale. South Pasadena, CA: Semiotext(e), 2020.

Hoffman, Wayne. *Hard*. Maple Shade, NJ: Bear Bones Books, 2015.

Hoffman, Wayne. *An Older Man*. Maple Shade, NJ: Bear Bones Books, 2015.

Lee, Christine Hyung-Oak. *Tell Me Everything You Don't Remember: The Stroke That Changed My Life*. New York: Ecco Press, 2017.

Manguso, Sarah. *Ongoingness: The End of a Diary*. Minneapolis: Graywolf Press, 2015.

McCallum, E. L., and Mikko Tuhkanen, eds. *Queer Times, Queer Becomings*. Albany: State University of New York Press, 2011.

Michaels, Eric. *Unbecoming: An AIDS Diary*. Durham, NC: Duke University Press, 1997.

Muñoz, José Esteban. *Cruising Utopia: The Then and There of Queer Futurity*. New York: New York University Press, 2009.

Nelson, Maggie. *The Argonauts*. Minneapolis: Graywolf Press, 2015.

Phillips, J. B. *Your God Is Too Small: A Guide for Believers and Skeptics Alike*. New York: Touchstone, 2004.

Puar, Jasbir. "Prognosis Time: Towards a Geopolitics of Affect, Debility and Capacity." *Women and Performance: A Journal of Feminist Theory* 19, no. 2 (2009): 161–172.

Schalk, Sami. *Bodyminds Reimagined: (Dis)ability, Race, and Gender in Black Women's Speculative Fiction*. Durham, NC: Duke University Press, 2018.

Sontag, Susan. *Later Essays*. New York: Library of America, 2017.

St. Aubyn, Edward. *Some Hope*. London: Picador 2019.

Wojnarowicz, David. *Close to the Knives: A Memoir of Disintegration*. New York: Vintage, 1991.

Jonathan Alexander is a writer living in Southern California, where he is also professor of English at the University of California, Irvine. He is the author, co-author, or co-editor of sixteen previous books. His nonfiction has been widely published, especially in the *Los Angeles Review of Books*, and his critical memoir, *Creep: A Life, a Theory, an Apology*, was a finalist for the Lambda Literary Award.

CPSIA information can be obtained
at www.ICGtesting.com
Printed in the USA
LVHW080933091021
700002LV00010B/120/J